Psychological Issues in Obstetrics and Gynaecology

Psychological Issues in Obstetrics and Gynaecology

Editors

Niranjan Chavan
MD, FICOG, FCPS, DGO, DFP, MICOG, DICOG
Diploma in Endoscopy (USA)
Training in Endoscopy (UK)

Professor (Addl) and
Unit Head
Department of Obstetrics
and Gynaecology
LTMMC and GH, Sion, Mumbai
Vice President, MOGS 2020-21
Jt Treasurer-Elect, FOGSI 2021

Avinash De Sousa
DPM, MPhil (Psychology), MS

Research Associate
Department of Psychiatry
LTMMC and GH
Sion, Mumbai
Founder Trustee: De Sousa
Foundation

Komal Chavan
MD, DNB, MNAMS, FCPS, DGO, FICOG
Diploma in Reproductive Medicine
(UKSH Germany)

Asst. Honorary Professor
Department of Obstetrics and
Gynaecology
HBT Medical College and RN
Cooper Hospital
Juhu, Mumbai

Co-Editors

Sneha Venkateswaran
MS (Obstetrics and Gynaecology)
Speciality Medical Officer
Department of Obstetrics and
Gynaecology
LTMMC and GH
Sion, Mumbai

Meenakshi Ruhil
MS (Obstetrics and Gynaecology)
Speciality Medical Officer
Department of Obstetrics and
Gynaecology
LTMMC and GH
Sion, Mumbai

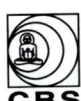

CBS

CBS Publishers & Distributors Pvt Ltd

New Delhi • Bengaluru • Chennai • Kochi • Kolkata • Mumbai
Hyderabad • Jharkhand • Nagpur • Patna • Pune • Uttarakhand

Psychological Issues in Obstetrics and Gynaecology

ISBN: 978-93-89565-91-1

Copyright © Editors and Publisher

First Edition: 2021

Published by Satish Kumar Jain and produced by Varun Jain for

CBS Publishers & Distributors Pvt Ltd

4819/XI Prahlad Street, 24 Ansari Road, Daryaganj, New Delhi 110 002, India
Ph: 011-23289259, 23266861, 23266867   Fax: 011-23243014   Website: www.cbspd.com
                                                                  e-mail: delhi@cbspd.com; cbspubs@airtelmail.in.
Corporate Office: 204 FIE, Industrial Area, Patparganj, Delhi 110 092
Ph: 011-4934 4934   Fax: 011-4934 4935   e-mail: publishing@cbspd.com; publicity@cbspd.com

Branches

• **Bengaluru:** Seema House 2975, 17th Cross, K.R. Road,
  Banasankari 2nd Stage, Bengaluru 560 070, Karnataka, India
  Ph: +91-80-26771678/79   Fax: +91-80-26771680   e-mail: bangalore@cbspd.com
• **Chennai:** 7, Subbaraya Street, Shenoy Nagar, Chennai 600 030, Tamil Nadu, India
  Ph: +91-44-26680620, 26681266   Fax: +91-44-42032115   e-mail: chennai@cbspd.com
• **Kochi:** 42/1325, 1326, Power House Road, Opp KSEB, Power House, Ernakulam 682 018, Kochi, Kerala, India
  Ph: +91-484-4059061-67   Fax: +91-484-4059065   e-mail: kochi@cbspd.com
• **Kolkata:** 6/B, Ground Floor, Rameswar Shaw Road, Kolkata-700 014, West Bengal, India
  Ph: +91-33-22891126, 22891127, 22891128   e-mail: kolkata@cbspd.com
• **Mumbai:** 83-C, Dr E Moses Road, Worli, Mumbai-400018, Maharashtra, India
  Ph: +91-22-24902340/41   Fax: +91-22-24902342   e-mail: mumbai@cbspd.com

Representatives

• **Hyderabad**   0-9885175004   • **Jharkhand**   0-9811541605   • **Nagpur**   0-9421945513   • **Patna**   0-9334159340
• **Pune**   0-9623451994   • **Uttarakhand**   0-9716462459

Printed at Goyal Offset Works (P) Limited, India

List of Contributors

Ashwini Bhalerao Gandhi
MD, DGO, DNB, DFP, FCPS, FICOG, MICOG
Consultant Gynaecologist
PD Hinduja National Hospital
and Medical Research
Center, Mumbai
Past President, MOGS
Past Vice President, FOGSI

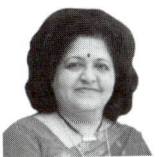

Avinash De Sousa
DPM, MPhil (Psychology), MS
Research Associate
Department of Psychiatry
LTMMC and GH
Sion, Mumbai
Founder Trustee: De Sousa
Foundation

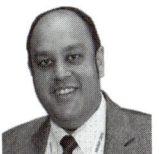

Hrishikesh Pai
MD, MSc, FRCOG, FCPS, FICOG
Consultant IVF Specialist
Lilavati Hospital, Mumbai
Medical Director
Bloom IVF Group
Past President, MOGS
President Elect FOGSI 2022

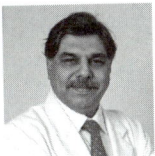

Komal Chavan
MD, DNB, MNAMS, FCPS, DGO, FICOG
Asst. Honorary Professor
Department of Obstetrics
and Gynaecology
HBT Medical College and
RN Cooper Hospital
Juhu, Mumbai

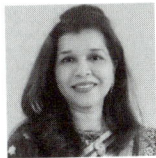

Meenakshi Ruhil
MS (Obstetrics and Gynaecology)
Speciality Medical Officer
Department of Obstetrics
and Gynaecology
LTMMC and GH
Sion, Mumbai

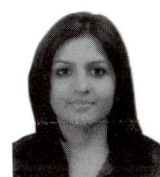

Nandita Palshetkar
MD, FCPS, FICOG
IVF Consultant
Medical Director, Bloom IVF
Center
President, AMOGS
Past President, FOGSI
IAGE, MOGS

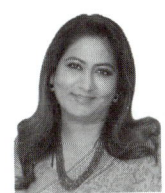

Niranjan Chavan
MD, FICOG, FCPS, DGO, DFP
Professor (Addl) and
Unit Head
Department of Obstetrics
and Gynaecology
LTMMC and GH
Sion, Mumbai

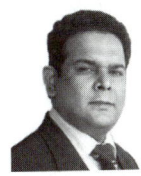

Priyanka Sonawane
MS
Speciality Medical Officer
LTMMC and GH
Sion, Mumbai

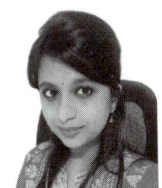

Ms Pragya Lodha
MA (Clinical Psychology)
Clinical Psychologist
Mumbai

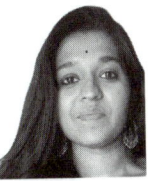

Rishma Dhillon Pai
MD, DGO, DNB, FRCOG, FCPS, FICOG
Consultant Obstetrician and
Gynaecologist, Lilavati
Hospital, Mumbai
President, Mumbai
Obstetrics & Gynaecological
Society (MOGS) 2020–21
Past President, FOGSI, IAGE, ISAR

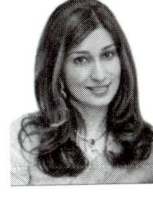

Rohan Palshetkar
MS, FRM
ART Consultant and
Endoscopic Surgeon
Assistant Professor
Department of Obstetrics
and Gynaecology
Dr DY Patil Medical College
and Hospital, Navi Mumbai
Head of Unit of Bloom IVF, Nerul

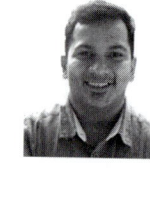

Sneha Venkateswaran
MS (Obstetrics and Gynaecology)
Speciality Medical Officer
Department of Obstetrics
and Gynaecology
LTMMC and GH
Sion, Mumbai

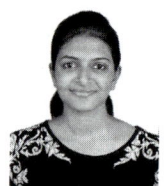

Sushma Sonavane
MD (Psychiatry)
Professor
Department of Psychiatry
LTMMC and GH
Sion, Mumbai

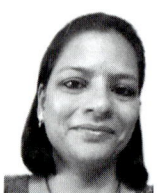

Ms Tejasvi Dave
MA (Psychology)
Clinical Psychologist
Department of Psychiatry
LTMMC and GH
Sion, Mumbai

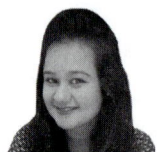

Foreword

It gives me great pleasure to write the Foreword for this one of its kind book which has importance both clinically and at a postgraduate level. This is a book that looks at the interface and interaction between psychiatry and obstetrics and gynaecology. There are multiple areas where there is an overlap between these two domains. The book has a large number of chapters that have been 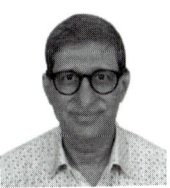 written by both gynaecologists and psychiatrists where both perspectives regarding a topic have been described. The book shall be appreciated by clinicians, resident doctors and academicians and at the same time shall serve as a primer for those interested in consultation liaison issues between psychiatry, obstetrics and gynaecology.

Prof (Dr) Nilesh Shah MD, DPM, DNB
Professor and Head
Department of Psychiatry
Lokmanya Tilak Municipal Medical College
Mumbai

Past President, Bombay Psychiatric Society
Former Secretary, Indian Psychiatric Society

Preface

The field of obstetrics and gynaecology is an ever-changing one. When a clinician fails to understand the psychological aspects of a patient's presentation, he or she is left feeling guilty of having provided substandard care. This book, *Psychological Issues in Obstetrics and Gynaecology*, explores the psychological issues faced by women in various stages of their lives. The book attempts to bridge the gaps in basic and specialist medical training in these issues. It is divided into five sections covering various obstetric and gynaecologic ailments and their associated psychological issues. It provides a complete yet concise guide to the risk factors, clinical presentation, diagnosis and treatment of these issues. It will prove handy for the consultant psychiatrist, obstetrician–gynaecologist, and a reference book for postgraduate students of obstetrics and gynaecology and psychiatry.

Niranjan Chavan
Avinash De Sousa
Komal Chavan

Contents

LIST OF ABBREVIATIONS

ABM	Academy of Breastfeeding Medicine
AD	Alzheimer's Disease
AED	Anti-epileptic Drug
AMH	Anti-Müllerian Hormone
BMI	Body Mass Index
CBT	Cognitive Behaviour Therapy
CE	Catamenial Epilepsy
DHA	Docosahexaenoic Acid
DSM	Diagnostic and Statistics Manual of Mental Disorders
DUB	Dysfunctional Uterine Bleeding
ECT	Electroconvulsive Therapy
FHS	Foetal Heart Sounds Foetal Hydantoin Syndrome
FSH	Follicle Stimulating Hormone
GABA	Gamma Amino Butyric Acid
ICD	International Statistical Classification of Diseases
ICSI	Intracytoplasmic Sperm Injection
IPT	Interpersonal Therapy
IUI	Intrauterine Insemination
IUS	Intrauterine System
IVF	*In Vitro* Fertilisation
LC-PUFA	Long Chain Polyunsaturated Fatty Acids
LGBTQ	Lesbian, Gay, Bisexual, Transgender, Queer
LH	Luteinising Hormone
LHRH	Luteinising Hormone Releasing Hormone
LSD	Lysergic acid Diethylamide
MCM	Major Congenital Malformation
MDD	Major Depressive Disorder
PMDD	Premenstrual Dysphoric Disorder
PMS	Premenstrual Syndrome
PMT	Premenstrual Tension
PPD	Postpartum Depression
PTSD	Post-traumatic Stress Disorder
SSRI	Selective Serotonin Reuptake Inhibitor
WHO	World Health Organization
WWE	Women With Epilepsy

Psychological Issues in Obstetrics and Gynaecology

General Considerations

Psychosomatic Medicine: Basic Concepts for Obstetricians and Gynaecologists

Niranjan Chavan, Avinash De Sousa

- In its simplest sense, 'psychosomatic medicine' merely indicates that there is a (psyche) mind–body (soma) relationship relevant to human health. Drawing from this, many non-professionals believe that it is a medical specialty that concentrates on the psychological influences on disease, particularly certain 'psychosomatic diseases'. Actually, it is a health science that is concerned with the nature of the mind–body relationship, including its clinical applications.
- More specifically, psychosomatic medicine is a field of health science based on the concept that the human organism is a psychosomatic unity, that biological and psychological processes are inextricably inter-related aspects of its function. This stands in contrast to the still predominant, traditional biomedical model from the nineteenth century which holds that diseases represent cellular or organ pathology arising from intrinsic defects or external biophysicochemical agents.
- Psychosomatic medicine conceptualizes diseases as occurring in persons, not their components, as a consequence of their transactions with an environment that is informational, social, and cultural, as well as biophysicochemical. It notes that people are not simply biological organisms, but sentient ones with motives, thoughts, feelings, and relationships.
- Mind–body unity should not be misunderstood to imply that mental and somatic phenomena cannot be separately studied. Such reductionism is a legitimate tactic that permits the study of scientific questions limited to that system. Each organ or part function merits study by techniques appropriate to it. To understand organismic function, however, requires a perspective that includes data from all body systems, including the psychological.
- Psychosomatic medicine provides no theories about the nature of the underlying processes. What it provides is its holistic perspective for interpreting them. It draws on the data, theory, and techniques of all other relevant fields, integrating these in unique ways informed by its conceptual base. Thus, contrary to common lay belief, psychosomatic medicine is not a medical specialty. Nor is it a scientific discipline. Its practitioners come from a range of disciplines and clinical specialties.
- Psychosomatic medicine is concerned with all mind–body relationships, giving equal importance to biology. Doubts have been raised about the aptness of the term. To some, the bipartite nature of 'psychosomatic' undermines the intended unity. But it is one, unhyphenated word. Others question the absence of reference to the social, noting that many relevant factors are such. Engel's alternative, 'biopsychosocial

model' was meant to resolve that, as well as to circumvent the residual misinterpretation that biology is devalued. But if social is included, what about cultural? Indeed, the list could include economic and other factors. Moreover, these factors can impinge on the organism only via the psychological apparatus.

- 'Psychosomatic medicine' also has the virtue of historical continuity that includes a mass of research documentation.

- Paralleling major biomedical advances that elucidated the etiology and pathogenesis of disease, psychosomatic medicine undertook a search for specific psychological causative factors. Dunbar was a pioneer here too, observing that patients with several medical disorders had distinctive personality traits which she concluded were aetiological. Others developed similar formulations. The identified diseases were termed 'psychosomatic.'

- This effort peaked with the contributions of Franz Alexander (1950). As a psychoanalyst, he focused on unconscious processes, but his work was far more elaborate and sophisticated than others. Most importantly and enduringly, he clarified that no purely psychological mechanism could explain the physiological processes of internal organs. Instead, Alexander reported that 'specific dynamic constellations' of motivations, defenses, and emotions characterized patients with each of a series of 'psychosomatic' diseases, and that life experiences which matched the vulnerabilities inherent in the particular constellation precipitated that illness. He also linked each constellation to specific physiological processes mediated through autonomic neural pathways that plausibly explained the pathogenesis of that disease.

- The brilliance of this work captured the imagination of many, and it became a major force in psychosomatic medicine. Belief developed that psychotherapy might cure 'psychosomatic diseases'.

- The evidence of correlations between psychological and somatic processes is extensive.

- When important meanings are attached to inputs, emotions are activated. These further affect body functions. The original response becomes a stimulus, too. In studying organismic function, what is defined as stimulus, and what as response, is arbitrary; it depends on what part of the process is being examined and at what point in time. Nor is this a simple chain of stimulus-response pairs. A network of actions follows, in which some responses affect one organ, some another, and some both, while some of these influences are stimulating and others inhibitory; and the succeeding responses become additional stimuli of the same variegated nature. Because many life events have more than one meaning, several such networks may be in process simultaneously. In most instances, then, a stimulus sets off a transacting web of responses and new stimuli with both psychological and somatic components.

- The endocrine and immune systems also serve as integrators of organismic function, directly and in their inter-relationships with each other and the brain. Pituitary secretions, which control many other endocrines, are themselves subject to control by hormones and neurotransmitters from the hypothalamus. Psychological stress is associated with stimulation of adrenocortical hormones via the pituitary, as well as neutrally mediated adrenaline release from the adrenal medulla. The distinction between neurotransmitters and hormones is blurred: Active neuropeptides and neuroamines are present in many peripheral organs. Hormones act back on the brain to inhibit their own overproduction, but also modify cognitive and emotional states. Stress also affects both cellular and humoral immune functions, partly through the action of adrenal steroids; depression may have especially potent effects.

- Psychosomatic medicine rests on the fundamental physiological concept of homeostasis: The human organism exists in a state of constantly dynamic equilibrium subject to both endogenous shifts and perturbations induced by an ever-changing environment. These trigger homeostatic responses which keep the changes from exceeding viable limits, thereby maintaining organismic integrity and permitting continuing function in the environment. If the change is excessive or the compensatory adjustments become so, damage results. When damage significantly impairs adaptation, disease occurs: Disease is failure of adaptation. At any given moment, every person is more or less healthy and more or less diseased.

- Psychosomatic medicine enhances this concept to take account of our inherent psychological and physiological properties as well as the sociocultural and informational content of the physical world. Moreover, although 'disease' may seem to have a fixed definition, different times, places, and persons have provided differing criteria for deciding what disease exists and whether one is sick at all.

- The application of psychosomatic medicine to patient care rests primarily on its basic concepts. As every patient is partly unique, only by identifying the issues specific to that individual can appropriate care be provided. The fundamental need both in diagnosis and treatment is establishing a trusting professional relationship that allows patients to relax defenses and reveal personal information and feelings. Also required are interviewing skills to facilitate patients' communications of their life experiences, along with physical symptoms and the life context of the latter. This must be accompanied by sufficient knowledge of psychology and social science to identify the significance of these communications, and also of major psychosomatic research findings in order to identify correlations likely to be significant.

- Treatment requires the ability to utilize this understanding of the patient in order to select the biological therapies that are most suitable for the individual, and to provide this in a manner that helps that patient use it best. On the psychological side, the need is to quantify and facilitate the extent of emotional release most helpful and tolerable to that patient, as well as the level of insight to pursue the relevant psychosomatic correlations. All this seems complex, and it is. But the knowledge and skills can be acquired in the course of existing professional education, provided that psychosomatic medicine is integrated throughout.

- This is true for all clinical specialties. As noted initially, there is no specialty of psychosomatic medicine. At the height of interest in psychosomatic medicine, a cadre of experts began to serve as educators of physicians, medical students, and others in academic health centres. Most were psychiatrists, although some internists and other specialists participated. This became a new subspecialty, named 'Consultation Liaison Psychiatry', as the service function became melded with education.

- But clinical psychosomatic medicine should not be confused with humanism or doing 'good'; it is applied science. Although its clinical practitioners act in a decent, humane fashion, it is not this but their skills and knowledge as applied scientists that make them effective.

RECOMMENDED READING

1. Fava GA. The concept of psychosomatic disorder. Psychother Psychosom 1992;58(1):1–2.
2. Fritzsche K. What is Psychosomatic Medicine? In Psychosomatic Medicine 2014 (pp. 3–9). Springer, New York.
3. Levenson JL. Essentials of psychosomatic medicine. American Psychiatric Publishing, Inc.; 2007.
4. Levenson JL. The American Psychiatric Publishing Textbook of Psychosomatic Medicine: Psychiatric care of the medically ill. American Psychiatric Pub; 2011.

Psychology of Indian Womanhood: A Commentary

Avinash De Sousa, Sushma Sonavane

INTRODUCTION

The conclusions of modern scientific research have established, among other things, the fact that many an old-world myth is an allegorical or symbolic presentation of the laws of nature which are basic to all creation. A significant case in point is that all nature is androgynous. Biologically, we have its analogue in the distinction between male and female. But the remarkable feature about this differentiation is that the component parts are not separate or disparate or mutually exclusive, but that each runs into the other interminably and inextricably.[1]

An indistinct, if not confused, echo of it may be detected in the Biblical version of Creation. According to it, God first created Adam and then, finding that he lacked companionship, took out a rib from his body as he lay asleep, and fashioned out of it woman to be his companion and complement. Mankind's generation was still a far cry, and, to account for it, Adam had to disobey God, commit sin and, as punishment for it, had to be expelled from paradise. This is the myth of the Fall of Man from a state of pristine innocence, and it is attributed to the frailty of woman his wife Eve! Here may be detected the germ of the idea of the superiority of man over woman, and it has been a decisive factor in, the shaping of Western civilization synchronously with the origins and spread of Christianity.[2]

The primitive Christian Church assiduously fostered this attitude, and to it we owe the twin phenomena of monasticism in its most extreme and bizarre forms, as well as a detestation of woman as the fons et origo of all human ills. So, we may say, without inaccuracy, that man not only exploited woman for his most imperious needs but, at the same time, gave her a bad name to preserve his own dominance inviolate! What is now known as the age of 'chivalry' was a breakthrough from such odious obscurantism to the opposite extreme of idealizing her into a goddess on earth, to act as a curb on man's predatory and libidinous instincts and impulses. What has uniformly eluded the grasp of the Western mind is the unalterable truth of their separate incompleteness. This is where our own (Hindu) concept of woman as maid, mistress and mother gives the picture in its totality a true and inspiring view of creation.[3]

MODERN INDIAN WOMANHOOD

A great deal of modern political and economic speculation is obsessed with the idea of inequality of the sexes with a reciprocal proneness for each to blame it all on the other, largely it would seem, to score a debating point here or there. Suppression, discrimination, exploitation and similar pejorative terms are handy missiles in this 'battle of the sexes' as waged in our own time. But the issues that are highlighted are, in the last analysis, peripheral and do not, indeed cannot, touch, much less change, the stubborn facts of nature. Chief of them is the obligation to motherhood which is squarely laid on the woman and woman alone.[4]

In none of our ancient records can we find any specific relegation or demotion of woman below man. She is the object of uniform reverence whether as child or maid or wife or mother. In fact, it is her crowning glory to be hailed and worshipper as mother. The Western idea of patriotism is foreign, if not repugnant to us. In our own case, it is Matriotism-worship of the mother wherefore we have made the earth itself our Mother and worship her in-protean ways. It has become intertwined with our religious susceptibilities as we may easily conclude from the decisive role this sentiment had played in our modern renaissance as well as in the national struggle for freedom. A detailed survey of our national history from ancient times would conclusively show that woman qua woman was never discriminated against. Rather she always rules whoever may reign. In all the annals of myth and legend, romance and recorded history, the unageing charm and varied appeal of woman and womanhood have nowhere found such puissant expression as in the heritage of India. Woman has played every part that man can, and has beaten him in her unique power to mother heroes.[5]

In Sita, we have the paragon of womanhood for the entire world and for all time. She is 'of the earth', but transcends both earth and heaven and stands as a symbol of vicarious sacrifice without ignoring or falsifying nature. She has inspired all the heroic women of our history in modern times, and her role has been to save our culture as often as it faced a threat to its vitality. Though frail as the trembling leaf and yielding like water, she is also Durga, the destroyer of all weaknesses and evils of life. She is also the creature of a new order out of the burnt-out ashes of the old, and thus renews life in perpetuity.[6]

THE CURRENT TASK OF INDIAN WOMANHOOD

To those who remember woman in a fit of absent-mindedness or uneasy conscience, a ritual tribute to her for one year might seem an appropriate amends. We have no such uneasy obligation cast on us because we celebrate her manifold powers in thought, word and deed all the time-consciously and unconsciously. It is the modern Indian man who is proving recreant to his trust, and poses a threat to our social and spiritual stability; and only our women can redeem him from his prodigal ways. 'Women's liberation', in our midst can only demote her from her regal throne to a level of equality with man which would profit neither, but would hasten the disintegration of her unique integrity. Both of us—men and women—have been rendered backward by the tragedies and ironies of our modern history; but even so, it is the restraining hand and indomitable will of our women that have helped us realise our frailties and follies. Her task today is to rediscover her Golden age in a modern context, and our duty is to create the conditions of her resurgence as the custodian of our culture.[7]

THE GAP BETWEEN FANTASY AND REALITY

Yet one must acknowledge that there is a large gap between the law and the social attitudes and beliefs which act as barriers against women's emancipation. Divorce remains at best a theoretical possibility, with the woman's economic dependence on the man in India and the social ostracism that a divorced woman suffers. Dowry has been outlawed, yet it remains a fundamental part of most marriage negotiations even today. Widow re-marriage too is in practice extremely rare. A widow, who put in an advertisement in the matrimonial columns, received merely three replies—as compared to the hundreds that others receive—all from men socially, economically and educationally her inferiors. And a recent study by a labour expert has shown that protective legislation for working women is actually beginning to work against women. Because of legal safeguards, such as maternity benefits and limitations on night work, employers are now reluctant to hire women. This has led to a slow but sure decrease in the percentage of women workers in the last few years.[8]

Indeed, the entire question of women's status in India is characterized by paradox and contradiction. On the one hand, we had a woman Prime Minister, women in politics, law, medicine, administration and other professions; on the other, we have widespread illiteracy, archaic rituals and an unshakable belief in the supremacy of the male. Again, there is a contradiction between the Mother India image, the Mother Cult and Goddess Worship and the other image of the Indian woman: Downtrodden, helpless, exploited and worn out to an early death. The lofty ideal of the feminine in Indian culture and the subjugation of women in everyday life is a continuing paradox.[9]

MALE DOMINANCE IN INDIAN WOMANHOOD

With most Indian women, the belief in male supremacy and female subservience is so deeply ingrained and so much a habit of mind that it never occurs to them to question it or to think about their own rights. From early childhood, they see the joy with which the birth of a 'son is greeted and the almost apologetic behaviour of the mother when she produces a daughter'. And so they grew up well conditioned to a passive acceptance of their lot; they do not resent it. After marriage, a woman goes from paternal domination to the role of the subordinate wife whose prime duty in life is to please her husband (and not annoy his mother). She is merely a biological mate to her husband; there is little companionship between them and they seldom go out together.[10]

Her security lies not so much in the love of her husband as in his regard for her in her role as efficient mother and housewife. In fact, she has no real status as a married woman until she produces a child, especially a male child. It is motherhood more than womanhood that we glorify, an Indian artist will prefer to paint a picture of a woman with a child at her breast and the Indian marriage still centres around the progeny. The Indian mother, her position being what it is, puts an abnormal amount of love on her son and expects from him "emotional fulfilment; an amplitude of life which should by rights come to her from mate hood only". This often makes it impossible for the son to have a satisfying relationship with his wife.[11]

INDIAN WOMANHOOD, CINEMA AND TELEVISION

This image of Indian womanhood is clearly reflected in Hindi films and in popular Hindi novels (on which most film plots are based). In film after film, the situation is similar: The wife is turned out of the house on the slightest suspicion and she goes away humbly, proves her innocence through all kinds of ordeals and timidly returns to her husband, who magnanimously takes her back. Sita-like, she braves all—from tyrannical mother-in-law to sirenish girlfriend, with never a word of reproach. Great emphasis is put on the hero's tenderness and devotion to his mother, whose will he will never defy, even if it means hurting his wife. Significantly, the heroine is hardly ever a career girl; if she does work, it is only as a supreme sacrifice to help the family tide over bad days. The Bollywood films also reflect a clear bias against the modern westernized woman. The vamp is almost always an independent type with short hair, who dances, drinks and is ready with the quick repartee, in contrast to the heroine, who would never dream of contradicting the hero or injuring the male ego in any way.[12]

SINGLE WOMEN AND INDIAN WOMANHOOD

The single woman in India has the worst of it, because socially too she has to put up with a great deal that is annoying to say the least. She has neither the freedom of the young unmarried girl nor the status of the married woman. Everything she does is misunderstood. She is treated as an object where men consider her fair game for any kind of "fun" they might have in mind. The single woman finds it difficult to take advantage of the city's cultural life. If they go alone to a concert or a cinema or a restaurant, they are often approached as though they were a pick-up and if they have a male escort, the gossip goes around that they are having an 'affair' with him. Others have complained of harassment from neighbours and from goondas on the street who are quick to seek out flats where girls are staying alone. While many working women say that they are not discriminated against in any way by their male colleagues, an equal number complain that they are not treated as equals.[13]

WORKING WOMEN IN INDIA

A common complaint of working women is that, despite their qualifications, interests and aptitude, they are always given 'women's work' because men feel women are temperamentally more suited to certain kinds of jobs, such as welfare or public relations. For instance, a woman architect says that clients often ask her to do the interior decoration of their houses, having asked a male architect to do the designing of the house itself, which is what she really wants to do. And a lawyer says that, at her association's meetings, she is invariably asked to type out the minutes, even though some of her male colleagues can type as well as she does. Because of preconceived (and thoroughly erroneous) ideas about the 'feminine temperament', when a woman loses her temper at work, men are quick to attribute it to "typical female instability and moodiness"; when she changes her mind on a particular matter, they say it is 'feminine capriciousness'. But when a man loses his temper, he is a 'disciplinarian', when he changes his mind, he is 'flexible'—both considered admirable qualities in an executive. A working woman is damned, if she does and damned if she does not. If she is assertive, energetic and competent, she is termed aggressive. And if she is quiet, unassuming and mediocre, they say she won't amount to much— what else did you expect from a woman? The married working woman, on the whole, has an easier time than her counterpart in the West, because she can still get domestic help. But if she cannot, then she shoulders a double burden, for rare indeed is the Indian husband who will help his wife with the housework or with looking after the children.[14]

NEED FOR A CHANGE IN INDIAN WOMANHOOD

Much is being talked, discussed and written about the different measures that have to be adopted to remove social and economic injustices to women. Nothing concrete has been done so far. Women must try to liberate themselves from their weaknesses and come out courageous as ever. Women should never hope that their emancipation would come through a man. True liberation has to be achieved through a woman only. Women who are detached, educated, able to teach, able to create their own scripture should rise up to the occasion to emancipate their sisters, without neglecting the uneducated rustic women toiling in the fields, tribals and backward classes ignorant of their own pathetic life, and the fallen women who are ill-treated for no fault of theirs. Women should understand that in everything simplicity is the supreme excellence. Women should never hesitate to protest against Indian cinema, posters and advertisements through which Indian womanhood is humiliated.[15]

Man and woman are complementary to each other. There are certain functions which only a woman can fulfil. Woman who is the giver of joy, inspirer of activity, maker of home and mother of children cannot do her part successfully, if she imitates man in every respect. While enjoying all the privileges in society, she should be careful not to misuse her position and transgress her limits. The vast and mighty ocean commands our awe and wonder because it keeps itself within its limits. Woman must realise the value of motherhood, sanctity of marriage, sacredness of family life and must contribute their best for the flowering of happier and larger family—our Nation.[16]

PSYCHOLOGICAL RESEARCH ON INDIAN WOMANHOOD

Despite the limited scope and impact of psychological research on gender in comparison to research in other social sciences in India, three areas of inquiry that are of crucial significance to women's lives can be identified. The linkages between work and family domains are of particular relevance for urban educated and middle-class women who have to juggle multiple roles in a context of diminishing traditional child-care support, inadequate state facilities for child care and, above all, stereotypical beliefs about the primacy of women's domestic role. It is being increasingly recognized that the key psychological variables mediating the work–family interface are attitudes regarding women's employment, and spousal and other sources of social support. The mental health profile of women shows that it is the category of common mental disorders that predominantly affect women. The aetiology and pattern of these disorders is indicative of the need to take into consideration the psychosocial and public health approach in contrast to the emphasis on the biomedical model alone.[17]

Another related feature is the gender-based inequities in access to mental health care, as a consequence of which women's mental health needs are either unmet or underserved. Research on domestic violence points to the interplay between sociocultural factors, such as the widespread acceptance of violence as part of marital life, and of male entitlement, the equation of masculinity with dominance and control over women, and individual factors such as low self-esteem, suspicion and negativism. As it is not only individual men who are involved in acts of domestic violence but also female kin such as mothers-in-law, it gives credence to the power and control thesis and the implicit mandate of the socioeconomic context of power relations rather than to male violence per se.[18]

Even so, this genre of research, reflective of a sample bias of the researchers, does not attempt to interpret the findings against the backdrop of the cultural valorization of women's reproductive and familial roles as primary which, according to the critical women's studies perspective, are delimiting factors in many women's lives. Mental health and domestic violence, on the other hand, are areas of research, emanating from the cross-disciplinary engagement between academics and advocacy groups and characterized by a critical women's studies perspective, calling attention to the existing power relations that are disempowering forces in women's lives. It is identification of this interplay between social structural and psychological factors that has implications for women's well-being and possibilities for meaningful interventions for enhancing the quality of women's lives.[19]

REFERENCES

1. Gatwood LE. *Devi and the Spouse Goddess: Women, Sexuality and Marriage in India*. Manohar Publishers, New Delhi; 1985.
2. Johnson RA. *Feminity Lost and Regained*. Harper and Row, New York; 1990.
3. Massey MC. *The Feminine Soul: Fate of an ideal*. Beacon Press, Boston; 1985.
4. Rae E. *Women, The Earth, The Divine*. Orbis Books, Maryknoll NY; 1994.
5. Stone M. *Ancient Mirrors of Womanhood Vol. 2*. New Sibbylline Books, New York; 1979.
6. Issac R, Shah A. Sex roles and marital adjustment in Indian couples. Int J Soc Psychiatry 2004;50:129–141.
7. Basu J, Chakraborty M, Chowdhury S, Ghosh M. Gender stereotypes, self-ideal disparity and neuroticism in Bengali families. Indian J Soc Work 1995;56:298–311.
8. Sharma I, Pandit B, Pathak A, Sharma R. Hinduism, marriage and mental illness. Indian J Psychiatry 2013;55:243–249.
9. Gadon EW. *The Once and Future Goddess*. Harper Collins, San Francisco; 1989.
10. Sangari K, Vaid S. *Recasting Women: Essays in Colonial History*. New Delhi; 1989.
11. Sangari K, Chakrabarti U. *From Myths to Markets: Essays on Gender*. Manohar Publishers, New Delhi; 1999.
12. Pandey J. *Psychology in India-the state of the art. Vol 1*. SAGE Publications, New Delhi; 1988.
13. Pandey J. *Psychology in India Revisited-Developments in the Discipline. Vol.2 Personality and Health Psychology*. SAGE Publishers, New Delhi; 2001.
14. Mohanty AK, Misra G. *The Psychology of Poverty and Disadvantage*. Concept Publishing Company, New Delhi; 2000.
15. Krishnaraj M. *Women and Development: The Indian Experience*. Subadhra Saraswat Prakashan, Pune; 1988.
16. Kapur P. *Marriage and Working Women in India*. Vikas Publications, New Delhi; 1990.
17. Davar BV. *Mental Health from a Gender perspective*. SAGE Publications, New Delhi; 2001.
18. Barnes BL. Mental Health Issues in Young Females: A Gender Perspective. Bombay Psychologist 1997;14(2):37–45.
19. Vindhya U. Quality of Women's Lives in India: Some Findings from Two Decades of Psychological Research on Gender. Femin Psychol 2007; 17: 337–356.

Psychological Issues in Obstetrics

Psychological Aspects of Abortion and Stillbirth

Niranjan Chavan, Avinash De Sousa, Meenakshi Ruhil

INTRODUCTION

This chapter presents information on psychological aspects of induced abortions, spontaneous abortions, and stillbirths. Stillbirths and spontaneous abortions are important maternal health indicators. Spontaneous abortion is traumatic event which can affect every woman differently. It can lead to grief, anxiety, depression or post-traumatic stress disorder. Globally, 12–15% of pregnancies end in spontaneous abortions. According to the studies, after spontaneous abortion, 30–50% may result in anxiety, 10–15% in depression that may last for 6 weeks. After a miscarriage, many women want information about why their miscarriage occurred, implications for future pregnancies, and support from health care professionals. Patient dissatisfaction often focuses on psychological issues.[1]

SPONTANEOUS ABORTION

Definition: It is defined as non-induced embryonic or fetal death with passage of product of conception before 20 weeks of gestation.

Classification of Spontaneous Abortion

Type of abortion	Threatened abortion	Inevitable abortion	Incomplete abortion	Complete abortion	Missed abortion
Pelvic pain	+	+	+	+	+/–
Os	Closed	Open	Open	Open	Closed
Passage of products of conception	–	–	+ (incomplete)	+ (complete)	–

Risk Factors

1. Age >35 years
2. History of spontaneous abortion
3. Cigarette smoking
4. Drug (alcohol, cocaine, excessive caffeine)
5. Medical disorders

Treatment

Threatened abortion is observed and uterine evacuation should be done in inevitable, incomplete and complete abortion. Management of depressive and anxiety symptoms after pregnancy loss can benefit future patient well-being.

INDUCED ABORTION

When a procedure is done or medication is taken to end a pregnancy, it is called an induced abortion.

The Medical Termination of Pregnancy Act, 1971

- Risk to the life of a pregnant woman or could cause grave injury to her physical or mental health;
- Risk that the child, if born, would be seriously handicapped due to physical or mental abnormalities;
- Pregnancy is caused due to rape (presumed to cause grave injury to the mental health of the woman);
- Pregnancy is caused due to failure of contraceptives used by a married woman or her husband.

Methods for MTP

1. *Medical methods*: Mifepristone (RU-486) and misoprostol (PGE1)—up to 9 weeks.
2. *Surgical methods*: Manual vacuum aspiration (MVA) at less than 9 weeks and dilatation and evacuation at 12–20 weeks of gestation.

STILLBIRTH

WHO/ICD defines stillbirth as the death of a fetus that has reached a birth weight of 500 g, or if birth weight is unavailable, gestational age of 22 weeks or crown-to-heel length of 25 cm. Within this category, ICD classifies late fetal deaths (greater than 1000 g or after 28 weeks) and early fetal deaths (500–1000 g or 22–28 weeks). The legal requirements for registration of fetal deaths vary between and even within countries. WHO recommends that, if possible, all fetuses and infants weighing at least 500 g at birth, whether alive or dead, should be included in the statistics.[2-4]

PSYCHOLOGICAL ASPECTS OF PREGNANCY

Pregnancy is an important event in a woman's young adult development that integrates femininity, sexuality, generativity, maturity, and future orientation. It alters the course of life of woman irreversibly, even if she chooses to terminate the pregnancy.[5] Depending on individual's personality, the normal psychological challenges of pregnancy can evoke a spectrum of responses, from maturation and resolution of old conflicts to decompensation and exacerbation of those conflicts (Table 3.1).

Psychoanalytic thinkers have explored the psychological changes in the women's life during pregnancy. Sigmund Freud explained as a girl's wish for a child as a 'substitution' for the wish for a penis, present in pre-oedipal stages of development. As the girl realizes she is 'castrated', her disappointment in her mother's inability to correct this deficiency leads her to expect from her father to repair this mistake. In this

Table 3.1: Normal psychological changes during pregnancy

- Increased introspection
- Preoccupation with the pregnancy
- Decreased emotional investment in the external world
- Heightened dependency
- Regression (shift to more primitive defenses)
- Altered body image

classic view, pregnancy for her serves a healing function, representing the ultimate fulfillment.

Freud's explanation of psychological issues of pregnancy as healing or repairing a deficiency has been softened and augmented by a more modern conception of pregnancy as a developmental phase that facilitates the transition to motherhood.[6]

PSYCHOLOGICAL ISSUES IN ABORTION

A review of the literature on psychological effects of abortion showed that when decision of abortion is taken voluntarily for an unwanted pregnancy, there is little evidence for long-term adverse outcomes. A transient feeling of guilt, anxiety, and depressed mood may occur, commingled with relief.

In a study by Freeman[7] of 106 women who underwent elective pregnancy termination, several issues emerged that corroborate the notion that the abortion decision is not a casual one. Thirty-seven percent of the women were studied who stated that they would never have considered aborting a pregnancy before their own pregnancy. Most women expressed ambivalence about the decision of pregnancy termination. Many found their decision and the time constraints stressful and felt isolated emotionally, unable to share their concerns openly with family and friends.

There are some factors responsible for negative psychological outcome after abortion (Table 3.2).[8–10]

In a Scottish study of 363 women undergoing induced abortions, 20% preferred medical abortion, 26% preferred vacuum aspiration, and 54% had no preference. Pregnancies with greater gestational age predicted a preference for vacuum aspiration over medical abortion.[11]

The women who expressed no preference were randomly assigned to undergo either medical or surgical abortion but no difference was found between the two groups in postabortal anxiety, depression, or self-esteem. Women with high levels of mood

Table 3.2: Factors for negative psychological outcome after abortion

- Past psychiatric history
- Young age
- Single
- Nulliparous
- Immature/conflicted relationships with partner and/or mother
- Involuntary procedure (fetal/maternal indications, external pressure)
- Denied abortion
- Medical complications

disturbance before undergoing the abortion, women who were smokers and women who experienced some medical complications after abortion were at highest risk for postabortal mood disorders.[12]

COLLATERAL EFFECTS OF ABORTION AND STILLBIRTH

Apart from the loss of a child, the grieving mother may also encounter collateral problems that can further deepen her psychological struggle in the aftermath of an abortion and stillbirth.

Marital Disharmony

Either or both the partners may individually experience grief in a detached manner which can cause a skew in the feelings of intimacy towards each other. Grieving mothers may feel guilty of experiencing pleasure from sexual activity and feel that she is betraying the deceased child. In such situations, the grieving woman may abstain from sexual activity for a significant period of time which can strain the relationship. The 'incongruent grief' of mothers and fathers may lead to frequent disputes and in a small number of cases, doubts about fidelity on the part of the partner may also be seen. The apparent 'emotional divorce' and withdrawal of intimacy can thus, succeed into marital disharmony resulting in outcomes ranging from hostility to legal divorce. Cases of domestic violence have also been reported as an extreme outcome.

Replacement Child Syndrome and Vulnerable Child Syndrome

Replacement child syndrome is achieving another pregnancy to fill the void of the deceased child by the affected parents. A variation of the replacement child syndrome is the *'vulnerable child syndrome'*, which refers to overprotective and controlling attitudes towards the subsequent child. Such a complex position may suggest the lingering of an unresolved grief for the parents and for the child, the possibility of having complex relationships with emotionally unavailable parents with subsequent attachment problems. The 'replaced child' may encounter developmental disturbances due to the consequences of growing with mourning parents and, therefore, struggle with forging a sense of self 'in the shadow of another identity'.

Following the death of a deceased child, mothers reported experiencing more problems with their living child as they exhibited more controlling behaviour towards him/her leading to strained parent–child relationships.

COUNSELLING

Preabortion Counselling

A careful biopsychosocial assessment of patient must be conducted, identifying high risk patients and those with already existing psychiatric illness. Interventions can then approximate the patient's needs more personally, maximizing prevention and thus minimizing psychological morbidity. First, a proper medical, gynaecologic, and obstetric history should be taken with a special focus on any complications or adverse sequelae associated with prior conditions. History of responses to stress and adversity in past from the caregivers should be obtained. History of any contraceptive use should be explored, assessing technical knowledge as well as psychological and relationship factors. Besides the painful emotional impact of a caregiver's obvious repugnance, such behaviour may alienate the patient and cause her to delay the procedure. Such a delay imposes the risk of a termination late in pregnancy or an undesired pregnancy to continue till term, with attendant morbidity to both the patient and her unborn child, as described previously.

Next, the patient's psychiatric history should be explored properly (Table 3.3).

Current psychiatric symptoms should also be assessed carefully, including mood, anxiety or panic, and substance use. If such positive symptoms appear, they may be powerful factors affecting the decision to terminate the pregnancy. A psychiatric evaluation should be carried out for clinical and consultative purposes. Active suicidal and psychotic symptoms (hallucinations, delusions, thought disorganization) should be considered as medical emergencies and should be addressed in a psychiatric emergency room or crisis program.

Finally, the patient's social situation should be assessed, including employment, finances, primary relationship with the partner, family support, and social network. Once a thorough psychosocial assessment has been conducted, a final checklist of risks for adverse psychological outcome can be completed, and appropriate measures can be taken to address these risks.

The other component of preabortion counselling is the sharing of information regarding the procedure details and its follow-up. Medical information should be communicated to the patient and the relatives in layman's terms and repeated for clarification, if necessary. It is important to acknowledge the possibility that the patient may experience transient feelings of sadness, anxiety, and guilt after the procedure, commingled with relief.[13] 'High-risk' patients should be counselled about the possibility of other, more intense symptoms and must be advised to report such symptoms as soon as they appear. Patients seeking abortion may have a choice of a medical versus a surgical procedure. In addition to provide the information and advice necessary for the patient to make this decision, the physician may note the results of the Scottish study cited earlier.

Postabortion Counselling

At the time of the follow-up after the procedure, a careful assessment of psychosocial adjustment should be performed. Symptoms of depression and anxiety should be reviewed, specifically, mood, sleep, appetite, irritability, tearfulness, difficulty concentrating, panic attacks, rumination about the procedure, negativism, and hopelessness. The psychological impact of the procedure on the patient's partner and

Table 3.3: Psychiatric history
• Nature of illness (symptoms, diagnosis)
• Precipitants (stressors, losses)
• Concurrent substance use
• Suicide attempts
• Dates of illness
• Duration of episode
• Inpatient treatment (length of stay, medications, electroconvulsive therapy, efficacy)
• Pharmacologic treatment (medications, doses, duration, efficacy, side effects)
• Psychotherapy (type, duration, efficacy)

family should be explored, in addition to thoughts or questions about future pregnancies.

In all interactions, empathic listening and a non-judgmental advice to the patient are essential components of the doctor–patient relationship. The best possible psychological results can be obtained in cases of abortion and stillbirths by having a good doctor–patient relationship by means of proper communication and counselling of the patient and the relatives.

REFERENCES

1. Kong GWS, Lok IH, Lam PM, et al. Conflicting perceptions between health care professionals and patients on the psychological morbidity following miscarriage. Aust N Z J ObstetGynaecol. 2010;50(6):562–67.
2. World Health Organization. World Health Organization; Geneva: 2006. Neonatal and perinatal mortality country, regional and global estimates.
3. Lawn JE, Yakoob MY, Haws RA, Soomro T, Darmstadt GL, Bhutta ZA. 3.2 million stillbirths: Epidemiology and overview of the evidence review. BMC Pregnancy Childbirth 2009; 9(Suppl. 1):S2.
4. Lawn J, Gravett M, Nunes T, Rubens C, Stanton C.The GAPPS Review Group Global report on preterm birth and stillbirth (1 of 7): Definitions, description of the burden and opportunities to improve data. BMC Pregnancy Childbirth. 2010; 10(Suppl. 1):S1.
5. Phillip DA, Carr ML. Normal and medically complicated pregnancies. In: Stewart D, Stotland N (eds). Psychological Aspects of Women's Health Care. Washington, DC: APA Press, 2001:13–18.
6. Fenster S, Phillips SB, Rappoport ER. The Therapist's Pregnancy: Intrusion in the Analytic Space, p2. Hillsdale, NJ: Analytic Press, 1986.
7. Freeman E. Abortion: Subjective attitudes and feelings. Fam PlannPerspect 10: 150–155, 1978.
8. Leon I. When a Baby Dies, pp 63–64. New Haven: Yale University Press, 1990.
9. Dagg PKB. The psychological sequelae of therapeutic abortion-Denied and completed. Am J Psychiatry 148: 578–85, 1991.
10. Blumenthal S. Psychiatric consequences of abortion: Overview of research findings. In: Scotland NL (ed). Psychiatric Aspects of Abortion, pp. 17–37. Washington, DC: American Psychiatric Press, 1991.
11. Henshaw RC, Najii SA, Russell IT, et al. Comparison of medical abortion with surgical vacuum aspiration: Women's preference and acceptability of treatment. Br Med J 307: 714–17, 1993.
12. Henshaw RC, et al. Psychological responses following medical abortion (using mifepristone and gemeprost) and surgical vacuum aspiration. Acta ObstetGynecolScand 73: 812–18, 1994.
13. Blumberg BD, Golbus MS, Hanson KH. The psychological sequelae of abortion performed for a genetic indication. Am J ObstetGynecol 22:799–807,1975.

Epilepsy and Pregnancy

Niranjan Chavan, Avinash De Sousa, Sneha Venkateswaran

INTRODUCTION

- Epilepsy is one of the most common neurological diseases worldwide. Women with epilepsy (WWE) are a common occurrence. Many of these women are in their reproductive years, and some of them may be pregnant and consume anticonvulsant medications.
- Epilepsy and pregnancy interact in a complicated way. The physiological changes that occur to maintain homeostasis continue throughout pregnancy and the new hormonal balance has the potential of altering neuronal excitability and the seizure threshold.
- It is well known that anticonvulsant/antiepileptic drugs (AEDs) interact with female sex hormones (endogenous as well as exogenous) by decreasing their levels. These pharmacological agents may also induce major malformations in the fetus. The teratogenic effects of these drugs indeed pose a serious concern for the patients and their healthcare providers.
- Although most pregnancies remain uneventful in epileptic patients, some may present devastating complications. This chapter shall provide an overview of various aspects of epilepsy and pregnancy.

EPILEPSY AND PREGNANCY

- A few prospective cohort studies have been conducted that show that there is no change in seizure frequency during pregnancy in the majority of WWE. However, the seizures may become more frequent in some (15–37% of epileptic women).
- Not much is known with certainty as to why some women experience increased seizure frequency during pregnancy. However, some factors that include sleep deprivation, altered anti-epileptic drug (AED) pharmacokinetics, or poor adherence to treatment may play a role.
- It was also found that women with focal onset epilepsy or those who were undergoing polytherapy experienced increased seizure frequency during pregnancy. During and immediately after labour, there is also a relatively increased risk of seizures (postpartum).
- Women who have catamenial epilepsy (CE) (epilepsy which is perimenstrual) have been shown to have a better seizure control, during pregnancy as compared to those who do not have CE.

Obstetric Complications with Epilepsy and Pregnancy

- Although most WWE have healthy pregnancies, they are still considered to be at an increased risk of suffering from pregnancy-related complications. This risk is higher when WWE are also on AED therapy. A pregnancy registry from India has shown that WWE are more likely to have spontaneous abortions as well as anaemia, ovarian cysts, and fibroid uterus.
- Meta-analyses and population-based data from many other countries show a small but significant risk of caesarean sections, postpartum haemorrhage, and induction of labour with AED exposure.

Fetal Complications with Antiepileptics in Pregnancy

- Focal seizures including unilateral motor or non-motor seizures, or some generalized seizure types like absence, and myoclonic seizures do not have adverse effects on pregnancy or the fetus. However, they may have indirect but serious consequences, if the patient sustains trauma because of them.
- Women with epilepsy who experience generalized tonic-clonic seizures may be at a relatively higher risk of harming the fetus during a seizure, even though the absolute risk remains very low and the level of risk may depend on seizure frequency.
- It should be noted that the risk of experiencing major congenital malformations (MCMs) in the general population varies between 1.6 and 3.2%, and WWE who do not receive AEDs show similar MCM rates. Hence, exposure to AED leads to teratogenic effects.
- Newborn infants of WWE who are exposed to AED *in utero* may have low birth weight and may also be small in size for their gestational age.
- Studies conducted in European and North American countries have shown that such infants have higher rates of low birth weight, preterm birth, intrauterine growth retardation, and smaller head circumference at birth. These infants also have lower Apgar score at birth as well.

Teratogenicity with Epileptics in Pregnancy

- Apparently, teratogenicity is variable among many different types of AEDs. We will consider the commonly used AEDs followed by some of the newer drugs separately for this purpose.
- Carbamazepine is still considered as a safer option among the older anti-epileptics, especially when compared with valproic acid. A very recent network meta-analysis showed an increased risk of overall MCMs with carbamazepine. Some studies have shown that the teratogenic effect of carbamazepine is rather dose-related.
- The teratogenicity of phenytoin has been well established among clinicians for almost 40 years. "Fetal hydantoin syndrome (FHS)" is found in 11% of newborns who are exposed to phenytoin *in utero*. An additional 30% of such children express some (if not all) of its features. Infants with FHS suffer from intrauterine growth restriction and intellectual disability. They may also have facial dysmorphism, hypertelorism, depressed and broad nasal bridge with upturned nasal tip, prominent epicanthal folds, and wide prominent vermilion of the lips, digital hypoplasia, and irregular ossification of the distal phalanges.

- Phenobarbitone causes congenital abnormalities with exposure during pregnancy that varies between 2.9% and 6.5% in different studies. Studies showed significantly higher rates of MCM with phenobarbitone as compared with controls. Most of these malformations are of cardiac origin.
- Data from pregnancy registries and prospective studies have revealed a significantly increased risk of MCMs in the neonates born to pregnant women who consumed valproate during the first trimester of pregnancy. The most common types of birth defects reported are as follows: Neural tube defects, orofacial clefts, congenital heart defects, hypospadias, and skeletal abnormalities. The risk usually increases when the daily dose exceeds 600 mg/day, but the highest risk is when the dose is 1000 mg/day or above. The individual susceptibility is genetically determined, making some individuals highly susceptible even with very low daily dosages.
- Current data on humans suggest that lamotrigine is less teratogenic than most of other commonly used AEDs, including valproic acid or phenytoin. The International Lamotrigine Pregnancy Registry update reported a risk of 2.9% with 414 mono-therapy exposures.
- In many registries and meta-analyses carried out so far, Lamotrigine appears to be a safer option, and perhaps one of the least hazardous anticonvulsants than other commonly used AEDs, as far as teratogenicity is concerned.
- In humans, topiramate exposure has been shown to be harmful for the fetus in pregnant women. The data from pregnancy registries indicate that infants exposed to topiramate *in utero* are at an increased risk for cleft lip and/or cleft palate (oral clefts), hypospadias, being small in size for gestational age, and increased combined fetal loss. Some studies have shown variable rates of MCM with topiramate that ranged between 2.4 and 4.2%.
- Levetiracetam, clonazepam and zonisamide have all been associated with MCMs when used in pregnancy though to a much lesser extent than valproate. Zonisamide in one study has been reported to produce low birth weight as a complication.
- Limited data is available on the effects in pregnancy exposure and congenital abnormalities with newer antiepileptic like brivaracetam, perampanel and eslicarbazepine.

Management of Epilepsy during Pregnancy

- There are many misconceptions regarding epilepsy which results not only in a late diagnosis of epilepsy but also missed or irregular follow-ups in epilepsy clinics.
- Folic acid supplementation is recommended that all epileptic women and girls (with or without treatment with AEDs) should receive a daily supplementation of folic acid in a dose of 4–5 mg/day before any possibility of pregnancy. Folic acid supplementation is believed to reduce the risk of MCMs in the offspring of pregnant, epileptic ladies. Although the evidence to support this hypothesis is not strong enough (class III studies), the studies that have been conducted so far do not show any evidence of harm and, apparently, there is no reason to suspect that it is not effective. Therefore, this recommendation is still valid.
- The aim of managing epilepsy in pregnant ladies should be the same as in any other epileptic patient, i.e. the achievement of complete freedom from seizures. However, the management should start before conception or even before marriage.

- All women who are in their reproductive years, even if they are not yet married, should be put on the safest possible AEDs with monotherapy and the least possible dose. It is advisable to inform all such patients of childbearing age who are on any AED about the teratogenicity of these drugs.
- WWE along with their spouses should consult a neurologist. If a couple plans to start a family in the near future, they should be evaluated and properly counselled regarding the possibility of experiencing a change in frequency of seizures during pregnancy.
- They should also be informed about the possibility of their offspring having abnormalities that include anthropometric anomalies as well as teratogenicity, and its likelihood should be re-endorsed. If an adjustment is required in medications, then the clinician should discuss the relative benefits and risks of adjusting medication with the patient to enable her to make an informed decision.
- It is recommended that before conceiving, WWE should have an adequate seizure-free period of at least 9 months with a single antiepileptic drug in the least possible dose. It is prudent to start folic acid supplementation after marriage or after the first pre-marriage visit, in case it has not been started before. It is better to maintain a preconception drug level with which the patient is seizure-free and aim to maintain this level during pregnancy.
- Taking vitamin K supplementation during the last month of pregnancy before delivery is advisable for pregnant WWE on enzyme-inducing AEDs who face the risk of intracerebral haemorrhage in the newborns. The delivery should be supervised by an expert obstetrician and a neonatologist. In addition, a neurologist should also be involved as a member of the team providing care to the patient.
- There is an increased risk of seizures during delivery, which can be caused due to multiple reasons such as physical stress, sleep deprivation, hypoglycaemia, inappropriate AED dosage, missing doses, and co-medications. The routine AEDs that the woman was taking should also be administered in the labour room.
- It is better to obtain the AED levels beforehand to ensure that the drugs are in their therapeutic range. Parenteral lorazepam should be made available in the labour room and can be administered intravenously, if the patient has a seizure during labour. The selected patients may require caesarean section, if they are unable to participate in labour, e.g. due to heavy sedation.
- The respiratory efforts of the newborn can be sluggish, if the mother takes phenobarbital or other sedative AEDs during pregnancy. A neonatologist or paediatrician should be available to resuscitate the infant. Many authorities recommend administering vitamin K_1 injections intramuscularly to the infant, if the mother had received enzyme-inducing AEDs during pregnancy to reduce the risk of haemorrhagic complications in the newborn, even though the evidence supporting its usefulness is very limited.
- It has been shown that traces of maternal AEDs can be secreted in breast milk. Therefore, there is a potential risk that breastfeeding might negatively impact children's development. However, a recent prospective study showed no such effect. However, more prospective studies are required to be conducted to evaluate AED exposure in infants who are breastfed.

- The expression of AEDs in breast milk decreases, if the protein-binding capacity of the drug is more and vice versa. WWE in their postpartum period should be encouraged to breastfeed their newborns before taking their dosage of AEDs to minimize the flow of AEDs into the breast milk.
- It is important to get adequate sleep, which might be difficult during the early post-partum period as it is usually frequently disturbed at this time. This can lead to breakthrough seizures. Such mothers can be advised to use expressed milk to feed their babies during the night. Moreover, WWE are advised to be careful and avoid positions that can be harmful to the baby, if a seizure occurs while they nurse their babies so that they do not suffocate or drop the baby or fall over.
- Gender and age should be important considerations when choosing AEDs for epileptic patients. Patients' and spouses' counselling are very important for managing WWE.
- As most of the women are already diagnosed with epilepsy before they become pregnant, it is prudent to give the safest medications along with folic acid supplementation from the beginning, even before they get married.
- Monotherapy is preferred with least possible doses. All AEDs are potentially teratogenic, but some of them include carbamazepine, lamotrigine, and levetiracetam seem to have a better teratogenic profile. However, the decision regarding AED choice should be individualized.
- Normal vaginal delivery is safe with appropriate pain and adequate seizure control. The patients should also be supervised during the postpartum period as they may need titration of AED doses then.

CONCLUSIONS

- The clinical management of WWE on AEDs during pregnancy is challenging. The goal of treatment is optimal seizure control with minimal *in utero* fetal exposure to AEDs in an effort to reduce the risk of structural and neurodevelopmental teratogenic effects.
- Physiological changes during pregnancy alter the pharmacokinetics of AEDs, which may result in lower levels and seizure deterioration in some WWE, but therapeutic drug monitoring and AED dosage adjustment during pregnancy and postpartum can mitigate this.
- Patients should be carefully educated on potential major congenital malformation, neurodevelopmental outcomes, obstetrical risks, perinatal complications and breastfeeding while on AEDs. It is important to monitor WWE during pregnancy, and despite multiple complexities in the care of WWE, it is important to highlight that the majority of WWE have healthy pregnancies.

RECOMMENDED READING

1. Battino D, Tomson T. Management of epilepsy during pregnancy. Drugs 2007;67(18):2727–46.
2. Nulman I, Laslo D, Koren G. Treatment of epilepsy in pregnancy. Drugs 1999;57(4):535–44.
3. Patel SI, Pennell PB. Management of epilepsy during pregnancy: An update. Ther Adv Neurol Disord 2016;9(2):118–29.
4. Tomson T, Hiilesmaa V. Epilepsy in pregnancy. BMJ 2007;335(7623):769–73.
5. Yerby MS. Pregnancy and epilepsy. Epilepsia 1991;32:S51–59.

Postpartum Depression

Komal Chavan, Meenakshi Ruhil, Pragya Lodha

INTRODUCTION

- Postpartum depression (PPD) is a common complication after delivery, and has increasingly been identified as a major public health problem. Untreated maternal depression has multiple potential negative effects on mother and the baby's bond and child development. Screening for postpartum depression in the perinatal period is feasible in multiple primary care or obstetric settings, and can help identify depressed mothers earlier.
- Some mothers also experience a mild and transient syndrome called 'baby blues' which is a short period of experiencing low mood and worry, which lasts for roughly one month.
- "Baby blues" is a term used to describe the feelings of worry, unhappiness, and fatigue that many women experience after having a baby. Babies require a lot of care, so it is normal for mothers to be worried about, or tired from, providing that care.
- Baby blues, which affects up to 80% of mothers, includes feelings that are somewhat mild, last a week or two, and go away on their own.
- Postpartum depression (PPD) is a psychiatric disorder that may present as antenatal depression or may occur as a postnatal condition, after delivery. It can predispose to either chronic or recurrent depression, and has negative consequences for the mother, infant and family.

RISK FACTORS[1, 2]

- Previous episode of PPD
- Depression during pregnancy
- History of depression or bipolar disorder
- Recent stressful life events
- Inadequate social supports
- Marital problem

PATHOPHYSIOLOGY

- In the pathogenesis of depression, there is considerable evidence for a pre-eminent role for three monoamine systems: Serotonin (5-HT), norepinephrine (NE), and dopamine (DA). However, when it comes to depression during pregnancy as well as the postpartum period, there is a need for greater research-based understanding for pathogenesis (and treatment).[3–5]

- Though popularly known that pregnancy protects against depression, clinically it is not seen to be true. Women with a greater risk for depression (than men), global estimated prevalence of depression among pregnant women are 14–20%, whereas that for postpartum depression is 10–22%.
- In a small-scale study of women with previously diagnosed mood disorders, it was reported that lower levels of the hormone allopregnanolone in the second trimester of pregnancy were associated with an increased chance of developing postpartum depression in women already known to be at risk for the disorder.
- However, larger and a greater number of studies are needed to confirm the same. Many earlier studies have not shown postpartum depression to be tied to actual levels of pregnancy hormones, but rather to an individual's vulnerability to fluctuations in these hormones, and they did not identify any concrete way to tell whether a woman would develop postpartum depression. There is preliminary evidence about the role of low levels of oestrogen and progesterone in triggering postpartum depression that demands for greater depth of study for conclusive understanding.

SYMPTOMS

- Feeling sad, hopeless, empty, or overwhelmed.
- Crying more often than usual or for no apparent reason.
- Worrying or feeling overly anxious.
- Feeling moody, irritable or restless.
- Oversleeping or being unable to sleep even when her baby is asleep.
- Having trouble concentrating, remembering details and making decisions.
- Experiencing anger or rage.
- Losing interest in activities that are usually enjoyable.
- Suffering from physical aches and pains, including frequent headaches, stomach problems and muscle pain.
- Eating too little or too much.
- Withdrawing from or avoiding friends and family.
- Having trouble bonding or forming an emotional attachment with her baby.
- Persistently doubting her ability to care for her baby.
- Thinking about harming herself or her baby.
- Other symptoms include persistent significant weight loss, insomnia or hypersomnia, psychomotor agitation or retardation, fatigue or loss of energy, and feelings of worthlessness or excessive/inappropriate guilt. PPD symptoms also include mood liability, anxiety, irritability, feeling overwhelmed, and obsessional worries or preoccupation often about the baby's health, feeding, and bathing safety.
- Suicidal thoughts are found in as many as 20% of the women with PPD. These symptoms must cause clinically significant distress or impaired functioning that are not attributable to a substance or to another medical condition.
- PPD is defined as a major depressive episode "with peripartum onset" and is elaborated as "if onset of mood symptoms occurs during pregnancy or in the 4 weeks

following delivery". However, in clinical practice and clinical research, PPD is variably defined as occurring from 4 weeks and may persist up to 12 months after childbirth.

- Depressive symptoms that do not meet full criteria for a major depressive episode which are seen to continue across the year after childbirth, may still have substantial negative impact on mothers, children, and families and, therefore, may require intervention. The bottom line for clinical practice remains to treat symptomatology irrespective of timeline and full criteria being met.

DIAGNOSIS

- Postpartum depression is one of the postpartum psychiatric disorders that include postpartum blues, postpartum depression, postpartum psychosis, postpartum post-traumatic stress disorder and anxiety disorders specific to the puerperium. PPD is a major depressive disorder with peripartum onset, i.e. symptom onset during pregnancy or within 4 weeks after childbirth.
- The Diagnostic and Statistical Manual of Mental Disorders-5 (DSM-5) diagnostic criteria specify that ≥5 symptoms must be present nearly everyday for at least two weeks,[6] including either: (1) depressed mood or (2) loss of interest or pleasure in activities that are normally enjoyable as at least one of the symptoms. PPD is difficult to differentiate from the major depressive episodes that may occur generally in a woman's life, however, what is characteristic is that in PPD the negative thoughts are mainly related to the newborn, feelings of guilt or inadequacy about the new mother's ability to care for the infant and there is a preoccupation with the infant's well-being or safety severe enough to be considered obsessional.

TREATMENT

The treatment for postpartum depression is usually a combination of psychopharmacological and non-pharmacological (psychological and psychosocial) interventions. However, there is a need for greater research to understand optimal treatment and management of postpartum depression.

- First line of treatment for PPD is psychotherapy consisting of interpersonal therapy (IPT), which is effective in mild depression, and short-term cognitive behavioural therapy.[7]
- Second line of treatment for PPD is pharmacologic treatment. No antidepressant has been approved as category A agent for use during pregnancy and lactation.[8–10] Antidepressants are used when depression is associated with signs of sleep or appetite disturbances or psychomotor symptoms.
- A combination of pharmacological and psychotherapeutic management is ideal.
- Antidepressants such as fluoxetine, paroxetine, nortriptyline, sertraline, bupropion, fluvoxamine, nefazodone and venlafaxine have been found to be effective in the treatment of PPD.
- All lactating mothers should be informed about secretion of varying amounts of drugs in breast milk. Though neonatal exposure to such amounts has low rate of side effects. But long-term effects are unknown.
- There have been suggestions for hormone therapy in the form of oestrogen and progesterone being given to pregnant women with PPD symptoms.[11] However,

results are inconclusive for the double-blind placebo-controlled trials about the efficacy of the same in the treatment for PPD. Thus, greater needs for research are recommended for understanding the efficacy of oestrogen and progesterone as treatment therapies for PPD.

CONCLUSION

- As a result of the stigma, mothers are less willing to take medication and, therefore, more open to seeking psychological and psychosocial intervention. Though with little support from systematic investigation, existing research supports the use of psychological treatments, specifically interpersonal therapy, cognitive-behavioural therapy and psychodynamic psychotherapy as well as psychosocial interventions such as non-directive counselling.
- Randomized controlled trials of psychosocial and psychological treatments for postpartum depression have concluded to show that both psychosocial and psychological interventions are effective in decreasing depression and are viable treatment options for postpartum depression.

REFERENCES

1. O'Hara MW, Neunaber DJ, Zekoski EM. A prospective study of postpartum depression: prevalence, course, and predictive factors. J Abnorm Psychol 1984; 93:158–71.
2. Wisner KL, Wheeler SB. Prevention of recurrent postpartum major depression. Hosp Community Psychiatry 1994; 45:1191–6.
3. Harris B. A hormonal component to postnatal depression. Br J Psychiatry 1993; 163:403–5.
4. Harris B. Biological and hormonal aspects of postpartum depressed mood. Br J Psychiatry 1994; 164:288–92.
5. Hendrick V, Altshuler LL, Suri R. Hormonal changes in the postpartum and implications for postpartum depression. Psychosomatics 1998; 39:93–101.
6. American Psychiatric Association. Diagnostic and Statistical Manual of Mental Disorders, Fourth Edition. Washington, DC: American Psychiatric Association. 1994 317–91.
7. Nonacs R, Cohen LS. Postpartum mood disorders: Diagnosis and treatment guidelines. J Clin Psychiatry. 1998; 59(suppl 2):34–40.
8. Prozac (fluoxetine). Physicians' Desk Reference. Montvale, NJ: Medical Economics. 1998; 859–63.
9. Pamelor (nortriptyline). Physicians' Desk Reference. Montvale, NJ: Medical Economics 1998; 1889–90.
10. Tofranil (imipramine). Physicians' Desk Reference. Montvale, NJ: Medical Economics. 1998; 1908–10.
11. Stowe ZN, Nemeroff CB. Women at risk for postpartum-onset depression. Am J Obstet Gynecol. 1995; 173:639–45.

CHAPTER

6

Psychological Issues in Breastfeeding

Komal Chavan, Pragya Lodha, Sneha Venkateswaran

INTRODUCTION

Breastfeeding or lactation is characteristic to all mammalian species. The benefits of breast milk to both the infant and the mother have been well established. It is not without reason that the World Health Organisation (WHO) recommends exclusive breastfeeding for the first 6 months of life, meaning breastfeeding being the only source of sustenance. Here we view some of the psychological issues associated with breastfeeding.

MATERNAL BENEFITS OF BREASTFEEDING

There is sufficient evidence to prove that maternal mental and physical health is positively influenced by breastfeeding successfully. Some positive impacts of breastfeeding on maternal mental health are discussed here.

Breastfeeding mothers have reported less incidence of anxiety, mood disorders and stress as compared to bottle-feeding mothers. Although these were reported subjective feelings, they were supported by objective physiological findings like reduced blood pressure, reduced heart rate reactivity, a stronger cardiac vagal tone modulation, reduced cortisol response when faced with stress and higher quality sleep seen in breastfeeding mothers. These effects, in return, have been shown to have a positive impact on the mothers' response to external influences and interpersonal relationships. These effects have been shown to be the result of endogenous increase in levels of oxytocin in breastfeeding mothers. Thus, the positive effects on maternal mood and affect have been proven to have a physiological basis.

Breastfeeding also improves mother–infant attachment and mothers who breastfeed are shown to spend more time with their infants, to touch their infants more and to have an increased sense of secure attachment.

INFANT BENEFITS OF BREASTFEEDING

Apart from the numerous health and nutrition benefits provided by breast milk, it has been proven that there are a number of positive cognitive, intellectual, social and emotional effects of breastfeeding on the growing infant. Longitudinal prospective designs are used to assess the link between breastfeeding behaviour and children's cognitive development. In one such study, there was a positive association between measures of Bayley Scales of infant development and the duration of breastfeeding in the first year of life. There was improved memory performance and earlier language and motor skills. These cognitive benefits were also shown to endure into adolescence. Specific nutrients such as the long-chain polyunsaturated fatty acids (LC-PUFAs) are present in human milk but usually absent in formula. Two major LC-PUFAs, docosahexaenoic acid (DHA) and arachidonic acid (ARA), are involved in neurodevelopment. They contribute to healthy neuronal growth, repair, and myelination. Infants produce a small quantity of DHA during the first 2 weeks of life, but are then unable to produce sufficient amounts on their own until about 6 months of age. Thus, infant cognitive development is sensitive to the supply of LC-PUFA in the first 6 months of life. In line with the finding that breastfeeding impacts the timing of myelination—whole brain volume, cortical thickness, and white matter volume have all been found to be increased among children with longer durations of breastfeeding experience. Longer breastfeeding durations have shown less parent-reported antisocial and aggressive behaviour in children from 4 to 11 years of age. These effects on antisocial behaviour extend into adulthood. There were greater amounts of hostile (aggressive) behaviour seen in longitudinally followed adults of age 20–40 years who were not breastfed as infants compared to those who were.

SUMMARY OF PSYCHOLOGICAL EFFECTS OF BREASTFEEDING

Lactation provides the optimal nutrition system from mothers to their offsprings. Research shows that there are psychological effects of breastfeeding on the child as well as on the mother (Table 6.1).

Effects on Children

1. Research data shows that cognitive development and emotional outcomes are generally better among children who have been breastfed. Improvements in memory retention, greater language skills and intelligence have been shown among children who are breastfed.
2. Research literatures have shown the long-term benefits of breastfeeding among younger children across adolescence and adulthood as well.
3. Initiating breastfeed right after the birth of the child has also shown to reduce the risk for cognitive impairment.
4. Mother–child attachment is enhanced during the process of breastfeeding that contributes to the overall emotional and mental well-being in the child.

Table 6.1: Maternal and infants benefits of breastfeeding	
Maternal benefits	*Infants benefits*
Less anxiety	Effective myelination
Improved mood and affect	Earlier motor and verbal skills
Less stress	Less aggressive behaviour (extending up to adulthood)
Reduced blood pressure	Improved memory performance
Reduced cortisol rise in response to stress	
Better interpersonal relationships	

5. Lack of breastfeeding has also shown to demonstrate emotional problems in adolescence.
6. Breast milk provides for PUFAs that are essential for brain development. The timing of myelination, whole brain volume, cortical thickness and white matter volume have all been found to be increased among children with longer durations of breastfeeding experience.

Effects on Mothers

1. Breastfeeding impacts the mood and stress reactivity among mothers. It affects the responsiveness to positive emotions in others as well.
2. Stress related to breastfeeding involves the mother getting up in the night, knowing when to breastfeed the baby on time, to know how and when the child is full or not, there is anxiety related to position for holding the baby, whether the quantity of the milk is enough. The Indian scenario also notices additional stressor due to the dominance of mother-in-law regarding the breastfeeding practices.
3. Formula feeding versus breastfeeding mothers show differences—breastfeeding mothers have lower cortisol levels and thus better respond to social stress, they have better sleeping patterns, form better social relationships and are overall happier than mothers who formula feed their baby.
4. Another health risk to keep in mind for breastfeeding mothers is that if breast milk is not removed, it can lead to the formation of breast abscesses which psychologically affects the mother.
5. Karl Abraham speaks of repugnance that mothers feel towards breastfeeding as they experience pain due to the baby biting the mother while breastfeeding. Medically, discomfort or pain in the nipples for 10 days is normative, however, prolonged pain must be got checked for. Sometimes, there may be some benign infections that the mother may develop during breastfeeding which are treatable.
6. Research has shown that mothers who breastfeed their babies are found to have significantly lower scores on measures of postpartum depression. It has also been found that mothers who have postpartum depression breastfeed their babies less. Additionally, it has also been found that breastfeeding reduces the depression levels in mother with postpartum depression.
7. Breastfeeding suffers when the mother may have medical issues and may be in the ICU and gets separated from the baby.
8. If on certain medication, mothers may not be able to breastfeed their babies and this psychologically affects the mother.
9. Breastfeeding is the process through which the first attachment takes place for the mother–child. Several mothers have reported that they want to breastfeed the child immediately after childbirth so as to establish the first attachment.
10. The breast being a vital organ of beauty for women, breastfeeding can sometimes bring body image issues among women where the mother and sometimes fathers feel that the process of breastfeeding leads to sagging breasts or breastfeeding adversely affecting the shape of breasts. Women report feeling not as beautiful which may also lead them to feeling anxious and depressed. However, this is a belief and finds no empirical evidence to support the same.

11. Women may want to undergo cosmetic surgery—breast upliftment and tightening procedures in order to feel better about their appearance.
12. Even when the child is unable to take milk due to medical illnesses, the mother experiences depression.
13. Problems of breastfeeding are seen in working mother where mothers experience guilt and sadness because of their inability to be present for the timing of breastfeeding.
14. Mothers often take to escape the breastfeeding process due to availability of formula feed, however, this leads to psychological effects on the child and mother (as discussed above).
15. In India, culturally, breastfeeding is an essential process and a moment of privilege. It is stigmatic for the mother, if she does not breastfeed the baby.
16. Some psychiatric medications can cause trouble for the mother while breastfeeding, e.g. risperidone can cause galactorrhoea.
17. Most antipsychotics and antidepressants can be safely given during breastfeeding to the woman and this must be clarified to patients as they often have this misunderstanding. It is suggestive that the last dose is taken after the night feed.
18. Another challenge is to make the child wean off from the 3 am feed as that may cause neurosis among the mothers.

BREASTFEEDING AND POSTPARTUM DEPRESSION

Breastfeeding behaviour has been linked to postpartum depression in mothers. It has been shown that breastfeeding mothers have lower scores on the Edinburgh Postnatal Depression Scale. They were less likely to be diagnosed with postpartum depression at 4 months postpartum. Another study revealed that depression in the third trimester of pregnancy was related to less chances of exclusive breast-feeding in the first 3 months post-delivery. Issues with breastfeeding may lead to earlier cessation of breastfeeding. Thus, early cessation of breastfeeding due to physical problems with breastfeeding may lead to negative mood and effect in the mother (Table 6.2).

Table 6.2: Common problems experienced by mothers while breastfeeding
Sore/cracked nipples
Breast engorgement
Inadequate milk production
Mastitis
Breast abscess
Improper latching method
Oral thrush
Blocked milk duct
Ankyloglossia "tongue tie"

Thus, due to the complex association between maternal mood and effect and the duration of breastfeeding, it is important to establish the exact nature of problem leading to cessation of breastfeeding. The cure for these physical problems are usually simple and give good results, and can potentially prevent the development of major postpartum depression.

BREASTFEEDING IN MOTHERS WITH MAJOR DEPRESSIVE DISORDER (MDD)

Maternal MDD occurs in 12–14% of postpartum women. MDD may negatively impact maternal breastfeeding intentions and practices. Depressive symptoms are associated with lower breastfeeding initiation, earlier cessation or both. Breastfeeding is interfered with because depressed women lack energy and miss infant feeding cues. Careful history taking and patient observation helps to diagnose whether the depressive symptoms are a cause or effect of breastfeeding issues.

Peripartum antidepressant use is seen in up to 8% of patients. However, the impact on prenatal SSRI use or maternal MDD on infant motor, language and social development has not been established. It has, however, been noted that women with prenatal depression and anxiety may show less intention to breastfeed. Patients with some sociodemographic characteristics associated with MDD (high BMI, low socioeconomic status) have shown to have less intention to breastfeed. These patients were shown to benefit from prenatal counselling regarding the benefits of breastfeeding to the mother and the infant. A multidisciplinary approach involving obstetricians, neonatologists and lactation consultants is helpful in this regard. Establishing breastfeeding support groups in baby-friendly hospitals is another way to ensure adequate counselling for mothers with depression from antenatal period onwards.

BREASTFEEDING IN MOTHERS WITH PSYCHOTROPIC DRUG USE

Several factors determine the passage of psychotropic medications through breast milk (Table 6.3). As the lipid content of hindmilk is higher, it is more likely that the drug gets excreted through the later part of the feed.

Drugs commonly seen to be used by patients with psychiatric illnesses are as follows (Table 6.4).

Selective serotonin reuptake inhibitors (SSRIs): SSRIs are the first-line drugs in depression, panic disorder, obsessive compulsive disorder and postpartum dysthymia. Neonatal withdrawal is seen with third trimester used of fluoxetine, paroxetine and sertraline. In lactating mothers, the infant dose is largely dependent on maternal plasma drug concentration. The effects in the infant seen with maternal use of fluoxetine are reported to be increased irritability, colic, decreased sleep, vomiting, and watery stools. Appearance of these symptoms in infants and neonates with no other probable cause for the same may point towards maternal psychotropic drug use. Overall, breastfeeding in women using SSRIs for various clinical conditions need not be discouraged as infant serum levels are found to be very low and of minimal significance.

Table 6.3: Factors determining the passage of psychotropic drugs to the infant through breast milk

Route of administration
Rate of absorption
Half life of the drug
Time taken to reach peak serum concentration
Volume of distribution
Degree of Ionisation
Water and lipid solubility
Molecular size
Plasma protein binding

Table 6.4: Summary of safety of use of psychotrophic drugs during breastfeeding

SSRIs	Moderate safety
Mood stabilisers	Valproate and carbomazepine considered safe
Antipsychotics	Clozapine is to be avoided
Sedatives	Shorter acting benzodiazepines are safe

Tricyclic antidepressants: Imipramine, doxepin, dothiepin, and amitriptyline are the drugs in this class. These drugs have a less favourable side effect profile and are best avoided in lactating mothers. Respiratory depression, drowsiness, hypotonia, poor suck and vomiting have been reported in infants of mothers receiving doxepin. However, it is necessary to weigh the risk–benefit ratio in trying to change the drug and dose when a patient requiring these medications is pregnant or lactating. If she has had clinical improvement in the past using these drugs, there is not much logic in changing the drugs during lactation as the change may cause poor compliance, poor response to the new drug and exacerbation of symptoms.

Mood stabilisers: Lithium is one of the first-line agents for use in bipolar mood disorder. There are reports advising use of lithium with caution in lactating mothers. Neonates are more sensitive than adults to the adverse effects of lithium. The adverse effects seen in neonates are: Cyanosis, hypotonia, heart murmur, electrocardiographic changes, lethargy, and hypothermia. The adverse effects in the neonate start appearing only after 10 days as that is the time required to achieve a steady state plasma level. Infants have a higher potential to rapidly get dehydrated and hence the hydration status, serum BUN, creatinine, thyroid function must be monitored in infants susceptible to lithium toxicity. Some authors recommend to use lithium with caution, and only if no other options are available.

Carbamazepine and valproic acid are not shown to have serious adverse events in infants of mothers consuming them, and are considered generally safe for use in lactation.

Antipsychotics: The use of clozapine and typical antipsychotics may be of concern for use in mothers who are lactating. Longitudinal data is lacking for recommending the use of atypical antipsychotics in pregnancy and lactation. In general, the use of atypical antipsychotics (except clozapine) like aripiprazole, risperidone, quetiapine is to be preferred over typical antipsychotics. This is a potential topic of research.

Sedatives: There is not enough data on the safety of use of benzodiazepines in pregnancy and lactation. However, as they are excreted in very minimal amounts in the breast milk, their use is generally considered safe. The shorter acting benzodiazepines like oxazepam, alprazolam and temazepam are preferred by most practitioners. Longer acting agents carry a risk of accumulation in the infant plasma. Hence, it is often advocated to restrict use of benzodiazepines on a short-term basis (1 to 2 weeks) (i.e. diazepam, midazolam, or lorazepam) rather than long-term use, as far as possible. Signs of sedation in the infant should be looked for.

Psychotropic drugs as a group are relatively safe during pregnancy and lactation. Women and their healthcare providers should not be unduly concerned, if a woman genuinely requires treatment. The clinician should be cautious about the uncommon but potential hazardous consequences observed among infants. Though there is evidence of transfer of most psychotropic medications through breast milk, drug concentration in the infants in most instances is less than the safety limit.

BREASTFEEDING AND THE WOMAN WITH DRUG DEPENDENCE

The healthcare provider faced with a pregnant or recently postpartum woman with a history of current or past drug abuse and desiring to breastfeed often faces a significant challenge for multiple reasons. Substance-dependent women frequently show behaviours or conditions that carry risk for the breastfed infant. There may also be direct pharmacologic effects of the drug on the infant. Drug using populations are also at high risk for developing human immunodeficiency virus (HIV) infection, hepatitis B and C infections. They may also be poorly nourished. Drug-dependent women who choose to breastfeed may be less likely to use or abuse the drugs in the future. Data from the1988 US National Maternal and Infant Health Survey indicate that heavy alcohol, marijuana, and hashish use and moderate cocaine use did not significantly alter the intention to breastfeed.

The Academy of Breastfeeding Medicine Protocol Committee has established a set of recommendations in the "ABM protocol" to recommend the suitability of women with drug dependence for breastfeeding. These recommendations help the healthcare worker to make a decision to either support, discourage or carefully evaluate the decision of the drug dependent woman to breastfeed.

Women who meet all of the following criteria under the following circumstances should be **supported** in their decision to breastfeed their infants:

1. Women engaged in substance abuse treatment who have provided their consent to discuss progress in treatment and plans for postpartum treatment with substance abuse treatment counsellor.
2. Women whose counsellors endorse that she has been able to achieve and maintain sobriety prenatally; counsellor approves of client's plan for breastfeeding.
3. Women who plan to continue in substance abuse treatment in the postpartum period.
4. Women who have been abstinent from illicit drug use or licit drug abuse for 90 days prior to delivery and have demonstrated the ability to maintain sobriety in an outpatient setting.
5. Women who have a negative maternal urine toxicology testing at delivery except for prescribed medications.
6. Women who received consistent prenatal care.
7. Women who do not have medical contraindication to breastfeeding.
8. Women who are not taking a psychiatric medication that is contraindicated during lactation.
9. Stable methadone-maintained women wishing to breastfeed should be encouraged to do so regardless of maternal methadone dose.

Women under the following circumstances should be **discouraged** from breastfeeding:

1. Women who did not receive prenatal care.
2. Women who relapsed into illicit drug use or licit substance misuse in the 30-day period prior to delivery.
3. Women who are not willing to engage in substance abuse treatment or who are engaged in treatment but are not willing to provide consent for contact with the counsellor.
4. Women with positive maternal urine toxicology testing for drugs of abuse or misuse of licit drugs at delivery.
5. Women who do not have confirmed plans for postpartum substance abuse treatment or paediatric care.

6. Women who demonstrate behavioural qualities or other indicators of active drug use.

Women under the following circumstances should be **carefully evaluated**, and a recommendation for suitability or lack of suitability for breastfeeding should be determined by coordinated care plans among perinatal providers and substance abuse treatment providers:

1. Women relapsing to illicit substance use or licit substance misuse in the 90–30-day period prior to delivery, but who maintained abstinence within the 30 days prior to delivery.
2. Women with concomitant use of other prescription (i.e. psychotropic) medications.
3. Women who engaged in prenatal care and/or substance abuse treatment during or after the second trimester.
4. Women who attained sobriety only in an inpatient setting.

CONCLUSION

As we have seen, there are many psychological issues associated with breastfeeding. These may be pre-existent or they may develop *de novo*. It is important to recognise the symptoms early, treat them adequately and counsel the women appropriately using a multidisciplinary approach so that the mothers and their infants get all the benefits of exclusive breastfeeding.

RECOMMENDED READING

1. Bayley N. Mental growth during the first three years. A developmental study of 61 children by repeated tests. Genetic Psychology Monographs 1933;14:1–92.
2. Cockburn F. Role of infant dietary long-chain polyunsaturated fatty acids, liposoluble vitamins, cholesterol and lecithin on psychomotor development. Acta Paediatr Suppl 2003;92:19–33.
3. Cooper WO, Willy ME, Pont SJ, et al. Increasing use of antidepressants in pregnancy. Am J Obstel Gynecol 2007;196(6):544–5.
4. Dennis CL, McQueen K. The Relationship Between Infant-Feeding Outcomes and Postpartum Depression: A Qualitative Systematic Review. Paediatrics 2009; 123:E736–E751.
5. Deoni SC, Dean DC, 3rd, Piryatinksy I, O'Muircheartaigh J, Waskiewicz N, Lehman K, et al. Breastfeeding and early white matter development: A cross-sectional study. NeuroImage 2013; 82:77–86.
6. Deoni SC, Dean III DC, Joelson S, O'Regan J, Schneider N. Early nutrition influences developmental myelination and cognition in infants and young children. NeuroImage,2018.
7. Dias CC, Figueiredo B. Breastfeeding and depression: A systematic review of the literature. J Affect Disorders 2015;171:142–54.
8. Drover J, Hoffman DR, Castaneda YS, Morale SE, Birch EE. Three randomized controlled trials of early long-chain polyunsaturated fatty acid supplementation on means-end problem solving in 9-month-old. Child Dev 2009;80:1376–84.
9. Fairlie TG, Gillman MW, Rich-Edwards J. High pregnancy-related anxiety and prenatal depressive symptoms as predictors of intention to breastfeed and breastfeeding initiation. J Womens Health (Larchmt) 2009;18(7):945–53. doi:10.1089/jwh.2008.0998.
10. Figueiredo B, Canario C, Field T. Breastfeeding is negatively affected by prenatal depression and reduces postpartum depression. Psychol Med 2014;44:927–36.
11. Gaynes B, Gavin N, Meltzer-Brody S, et al. Perinatal Depression: Prevalence, Screening Acwracy, and Screening Outcomes. Agency for Healthcare Research and Quality; Rockville, MD: 2005.

12. Groër MW. Differences between exclusive breastfeeders, formula-feeders, and controls: A study of stress, mood, and endocrine variables. Biol Res Nurs 2005;7:106–17.

13. Guesnet P, Alessandri JM. Docosahexaenoic acid (DHA) and the developing central nervous system (CNS)-Implications for dietary recommendations. Biochemie 2011; 93:7–12.

14. Hale T.W. Drug Therapy and Breastfeeding: Antidepressants, Antipsychotics, Antimanics, and Sedatives. Neo Reviews 2004;5(10):e451.

15. Heinrichs M, Neumann ID, Ehlert U. Lactation and stress: Protective effects of breastfeeding in humans. Stress 2002; 5:165–203.

16. Isaacs EB, Fischl BR, Quinn BT, Chong WK, Gadian DG, Lucas A. Impact of breast milk on intelligence quotient, brain size, and white matter development. Pediatr Res 2010; 67:357–62.

17. Kafouri S, Kramer M, Leonard G, Perron M, Pike B, Richer L, et al. Breastfeeding and brain structure in adolescence. Int J Epidemiol 2013; 42:150–9.

18. Krol KM, Kamboj SK, Curran HV, Grossmann T. Breastfeeding experience differentially impacts recognition of happiness and anger in mothers. Sci Rep 2014;4:7006.

19. Lavelli M, Poli M. Early mother-infant interaction during breast- and bottle-feeding. Infant Behav Dev 1998;21:667–83.

20. Merjonen P, Jokela M, Pulkki-Raback L, Hintsanen M, Raitakari OT, Viikari J, et al. Breastfeeding and Offspring Hostility in Adulthood. PsychotherPsychosom 2011; 80:371–3.

21. Snellen M, Galbally M, Udechuku A, Spalding G, Munro C, Drinkwater P. Psychotropic Medication in Pregnancy/Lactation. Revised 2nd Edition. Mercy Health & Aged Care: Melbourne; 2007. Pharmacy Department Mercy Hospital for Women. October 2007.

22. Tripathi BM, Majumder P. Lactating mother and psychotropic drugs. Mens Sana Monogr. 2010;8(1):83–95. doi:10.4103/0973–1229.58821.

Psychological Issues in Reproductive Medicine

Psychiatric Aspects of Infertility and IVF

Nandita Palshetkar, Avinash De Sousa, Rohan Palshetkar, Meenakshi Ruhil

- Involuntary childlessness has been a social stigma and has caused emotional trauma and relationship strain. The distress of barrenness impels individuals to seek a remedy, most typically a medical remedy, because realignment of social relationships is the least attractive alternative for individuals, couples, and communities.
- Infertility affects between 80 and 168 million people worldwide; approximately 1 in 10 couples experience either primary or secondary infertility. Primary infertility (involuntary childlessness) rates are 1 to 8%, whereas rates of secondary infertility (the inability to have another child) are significantly higher, at 35%. Compared with the middle of the twentieth century, when 50% of infertility was considered to be unexplained or attributable to psychosomatic disorders in the female partner (e.g. conflicted feelings about motherhood, her mother, or sexuality), today, 10% of infertility is unexplained, 50% is attributable to female factors, 35% to male factors, and 5% to other factors (e.g. both partners).
- Whatever the cause, most medical treatments for infertility are geared toward women, who bear a disproportionate share of the treatment burden. Global rates of infertility vary dramatically, from a prevalence rate of about 5% in developed countries to more than 30% in sub-Saharan Africa. The wide variance in prevalence rates contributes to the emotional experience of infertility; specifically, where infertility is experienced, impacts how it is experienced.
- "Stratification of infertility" refers to the barriers to infertility treatment which, understandably, impact the infertility experience and include economic, social welfare, and public health issues (e.g. poverty, malnutrition, obesity, smoking, and sexually transmitted diseases); ignorance of reproduction, sexual health, or fertility preservation; or lack of availability or access to high-quality medical treatments.
- Additionally, in many patriarchal societies (e.g. Middle Eastern and African), male-factor infertility does not exist; it is an unacceptable diagnosis, thereby increasing the psychosocial stress of male-factor infertility for men (because of the increased stigma and secrecy) and for women, who have few roles in society apart from motherhood.
- Medical treatments facilitate parenthood through assisted reproductive technologies, such as *in vitro* fertilization (IVF), intrauterine inseminations (IUI), intracytoplasmic sperm injection (ICSI), and third-party (e.g. donated gametes or embryos, gestational carriers, surrogates), to an ever-increasing range of individuals and couples seeking biologic parenthood (e.g. married or committed couples, gay or lesbian couples, or solo parents).

- In addition, reproductive medicine facilitates childbearing for individuals who previously could not have biologic children because of medical conditions that impaired their fertility (e.g. HIV/AIDS, azoospermia due to congenital absence of the vas deferens, and cancer). However, these new reproductive opportunities must be considered within the context of cultural, religious, economic, and legislative barriers that can, and often do, prevent couples from pursuing their procreative goals.
- Infertile patients are typically motivated to overcome treatment barriers by pursuing their preferred reproductive, family-building alternative where it is available and less costly. Some infertile patients are motivated by the belief that the level of care in other countries is better or preferable.
- With the advent of assisted and complex reproduction, the role of the mental health professional in the treatment of infertility has shifted from curative to a more complex and comprehensive role. Mental health professionals in reproductive medicine are expected to provide patient education, screening, guidance, and preparation for medical treatments; advice, support, and assistance with decision making; assessment of current mental health and marital and relationship stability; bereavement therapy; treatment of pre-existing or ongoing psychiatric diagnosis, sexual problems, or marital problems; and assistance with integration, transcendence, and recovery from the narcissistic injury and emotional crisis of infertility.

PSYCHIATRIC DISORDERS IN INFERTILE INDIVIDUALS

- Some degree of emotional distress in response to infertility or its treatment is expected and understandable. Reproductive failure or involuntary childlessness is a significant loss for men and women worldwide. Despite this loss, psychopathology is not a universal consequence, although some individuals experience exacerbations of pre-existing psychiatric disorders or clinically significant emotional problems.
- Frequent emotional responses to infertility include anger, guilt, shock, lowered self-esteem, sexual dysfunction, marital distress, and social isolation. Although most infertile individuals do not experience severe or clinically significant distress, sexual problems, or psychopathology, a small portion do.
- A recent review of the literature duplicated these findings, concluding that, although descriptive literature on the psychologic consequences of infertility presented infertility as a psychologically devastating experience, empirically sound research found no significant differences between infertile individuals and controls in terms of psychopathology or self-esteem. At the same time, infertile individuals undergoing assisted reproduction do appear to be at greater risk for psychologic distress (e.g. anxiety, distress, and grief), particularly if treatment is unsuccessful.
- Factors contributing to grief reaction following unsuccessful IVF/ET included a belief that the treatment is the couple's last chance at having a biologic child; pre-existing psychologic illness; and overestimation of personal success.
- Research indicates that mood (anxiety, depression, or distress) fluctuates in men and women over the course of assisted reproduction treatment cycles (anxiety and depression increase on oocyte-retrieval day, decrease on embryo-transfer day, and rise again on pregnancy-testing day), with the severity of emotional distress diminishing with repeated cycles.

- Although most individuals are able to manage the experience of infertility effectively, a small portion will develop serious psychopathology requiring immediate psychiatric care. In addition, despite a lack of prevalence or incidence studies, it must be assumed that some reproductive collaborators will also present with a current or pre-existing psychiatric disorder, or will develop one while participating in reproductive therapies. As such, it is imperative that all clinicians understand the potential effects of infertility medications, psychotropic medications, and psychopathology to provide appropriate psychiatric patient care; consult with reproductive caregivers about the risks and benefits of reproductive treatment for individuals psychologically at-risk; and ensure the emotional well-being of infertile individuals during and after treatment.

Observed Psychologic Effects of Infertility

A. Emotional effects
- Grieving and depression
- Anger and frustration
- Guilt
- Shock and denial
- Anxiety

B. Loss of control
- Loss of control over activities, body, emotions
- Inability to predict and plan future
- Loss of health
- Loss of security (about a predictable future)

C. Effects on self-esteem, identity, beliefs
- Loss of self-esteem and self-confidence, feelings of inadequacy
- Identity problems or shifts, loss of status or prestige
- Changes in world views

D. Social effects
- Effects on marital interactions and satisfaction (positive and negative)
- Effects on sexual functioning
- Different social network interactions, changes in relationships with network members, loneliness, embarrassment

E. Loss of a (potential) relationship
- Loss of fantasy or hope of fulfilling an important fantasy
- Loss of something or someone of great symbolic value
- Loss of future and past in one person

Psychological Responses to Infertility

- Depression
- Dysthymia
- Bipolar disorder
- Bereavement (complicated or delayed), pathological grief

- Anxiety disorders
- Obsessive/compulsive disorder
- Panic attacks
- Phobias
- Post-traumatic stress disorder
- Eating disorders
- Personality disorders
- Sexual dysfunction
- History of rape, trauma
- Low libido
- Infrequent or no sexual intercourse
- Anorgasmia
- Addiction problems
- Alcohol
- Gambling
- Prescription medication
- Tobacco
- Recreational drugs
- Sex/pornography
- Relationship problems
- Infidelity
- Sexual difficulties
- Anger management/violence
- Communication problems
- Lack of shared goals
- Behavioural problems
- Non-compliance with treatment
- Occupational problems
- Identity issues
- Legal difficulties
- Impulse control issues
- Religious or spiritual difficulties
- Acculturation issues
- Phase of life problems
- Sleep disturbances
- Somatization disorder
- Factitious disorder

Stress and Post-Traumatic Stress Syndrome

- Post-traumatic stress syndrome is an anxiety disorder that typically develops after a terrifying experience involving an actual or perceived threat of physical harm. For most, infertility is not a discrete event but an evolving process that initially involves a potential threat or loss, which develops over time into a real threat or loss (e.g. childlessness, repeated failed cycles or miscarriages).

- Infertility is stressful in that it is an unpredictable experience, which is negative, uncontrollable, and ambiguous. Further, anxiety during treatment and the outcome of the treatment itself appear to be associated, with both men and women experiencing substantial distress over time, especially when treatment proves unsuccessful.
- For most individuals, infertility and its treatment do not precipitate post-traumatic stress disorder (PTSD), unless they experience a particularly traumatic treatment outcome (e.g. lost embryos, medical crisis during treatment). More often, men and women enter infertility treatment with a history of PTSD that impacts their ability to cope and manage in a healthy fashion the distress of infertility. An example is the individual whose prior history of sexual abuse or trauma early in life triggers anxiety during infertility treatment (e.g. vaginal probe ultrasound, producing a semen specimen at the clinic).
- In these circumstances, caregivers may need to adapt treatment procedures, and psychiatric care may involve relaxation techniques or long-term treatment care, such as psychotherapy, to ensure that the PTSD symptoms remain manageable.

Sexual Dysfunction

- The most common female sexual dysfunctions in infertile women are arousal phase disorders; orgasm phase disorders; vaginismus; and dyspareunia. Sexual dysfunction in women may be due to hormonal changes, anatomic or physical factors (e.g. endometriosis, ovarian cysts, or uterine fibroids), or organic conditions (e.g. illness and diseases impacting general well-being and sexual health).
- Female sexual pain disorders can become the cause of infertility, if not the result, when pain is intense enough to limit or halt sexual intercourse. This situation is common in conditions such as endometriosis, uterine fibroids, perimenopause, and uterine anomalies.
- The most common sexual dysfunctions in men are erectile dysfunction, premature ejaculation, and retarded or inhibited ejaculation. Erectile dysfunction is the most important cause of male-factor infertility due to sexual dysfunction, although men rarely disclose this problem to caregivers. Treatments for secondary erectile dysfunction have had mixed success rates, although medications (e.g. sildenafil citrate or vardenafil) have been found to be effective. Additionally, sildenafil citrate has also been found to improve seminal parameters (e.g. sperm motility).
- Sildenafil citrate was found to be helpful in increasing compliance among men using intercourse to conceive or pursuing infertility treatments that required semen collection.

Personality Types and Infertility
Personality Structure Reaction to Infertility

- *Obsessive*: Orderly, systematic, perfectionist, inflexible—infertility is seen as punishment for letting things get out of control.
- *Narcissistic*: Self-involved, angry, independent, perfectionist—infertility is seen as an attack on autonomy and perfection of self.
- *Borderline*: Demanding, impulsive, unstable—infertility is seen as a threat of abandonment.
- *Dependent*: Long-suffering, depressed, submissive—infertility is seen as expected punishment for worthlessness.

- *Avoidant*: Remote, unsociable, uninvolved—infertility and its procedures are seen as a dangerous invasion of privacy.
- *Paranoid*: Wary, suspicious, blaming, hypersensitive—infertility is seen as annihilating assault coming from everywhere outside of self.

PSYCHOLOGIC RESPONSES TO INFERTILITY TREATMENT MEDICATIONS

- Oral birth control pills are typically used as part of the IVF treatment cycle to downregulate the hypothalamus, to prevent premature ovulation during IVF cycles. Prevalence rates of depression in women taking oral birth control pills range from 5 to 50%, depression being most common in progesterone-dominant pills.
- However, because of the estrogen in oral birth control pills, some studies have reported the induction of rapid cycling mood in women with bipolar disorder when taking these pills.
- GnRH agonists (e.g. lupron) are also typically used as a part of the IVF treatment cycle for downregulation of the pituitary, to prevent premature ovulation during the IVF cycle. When used during an IVF treatment cycle, GnRH agonists are typically begun in the midluteal phase of the preceding cycle and continued until the stimulation phase of the treatment cycle. As noted earlier, GnRH agonists can lead to acute hypoestrogenism, triggering menopausal symptoms.
- Researchers found that triptorelin caused a 40% reduction in oestradiol levels during the pretreatment phase, and this hypoestrogenism was associated with significantly increased symptoms of anxiety and depression, compared with controls.

Psychiatric Effects of Infertility Medications

Bromocriptine: Hyperprolactinaemia, antidepressant effects, hypomania, psychosis.

Leuprolide acetate: Hypothalamic downregulation, depression, cognitive problems, fine motor problems.

Progesterone: Endometrial support, depression, decreased libido, irritability.

Oestradiol: Endometrial support, antidepressant effects, induction of rapid cycling.

COLLABORATION WITH THE REPRODUCTIVE MEDICINE TEAM

- Some infertility clinics recommend or require that patients inform all caregivers (e.g. psychiatrist or any other medicating physician) that he/she is undergoing infertility treatment. This requirement improves patient care (e.g. reducing the potential for drug interactions) and reinforces a collaborative approach to infertility treatment.
- This collaboration is even more important when the patient also has complicating medical conditions for which he/she is being treated with other medications. Infertile individuals, however, may not be forthcoming with reproductive medicine caregivers about their current or past psychiatric problems because of ignorance (i.e. lack of awareness of the potential for drug interactions); a belief that mental and physical health problems are two separate problems; embarrassment about the psychologic diagnosis; fear that infertility treatment will be denied or postponed because of the mental health problem and diagnosis; or denial, a belief that they (or their partner) does not have a mental health problem. Ideally, decisions about psychotropic medication usage and reproduction are made collaboratively and

openly with the patient (and partner) as educated participants in the decision-making process with a reproductive psychiatrist.

- With the patient's permission, these decisions should be promptly communicated to the reproductive medicine team including on staff infertility counselor(s). The plan should address setbacks, whether mental health or medical (e.g. failed treatment cycle); crisis intervention; and pregnancy. Given that infertile men and women are known to be psychologically and physically vulnerable individually, as a couple, and as potential parents, it is imperative that the psychiatric needs of infertile patients be recognized and proactively addressed. Increasingly, psychiatrists work either as infertility counselors or with infertility counselors to improve the care and well-being of men and women undergoing infertility treatment.

- Psychiatrists, particularly those who provide primarily psychopharmacologic care, may or may not be aware that their patient is infertile; a gamete donor; a surrogate; pursuing pregnancy; or taking reproductive treatment medications.

- Psychiatrists are typically called on by the reproductive medicine team to evaluate psychiatric readiness for medical procedures (e.g. IVF, gamete donation); treat a patient who has an active psychiatric disorder or a history of psychopathology, or who is on psychotropic medications; and assess a patient's mental status (e.g. ability to provide informed consent). Input from psychiatrists is particularly important with regard to decisions about denial of treatment or participation as a reproductive helper because of confounding mental health diagnosis or psychopharmacologic contraindications. They are in the best position to educate patients about the side effects of infertility treatment medications and the impact of hormonal shifts on psychologic well-being, particularly if the individual has pre-existing or ongoing psychopathology. They can be helpful with differential diagnosis among grief, depression, and stress; in assessing psychologic preparedness; and in determining the acceptability and suitability of gamete donation, a gestational carrier, or surrogacy as a family-building alternative for individuals, couples, and reproductive collaborators.

- Psychiatrists can also be helpful when considering the long-term psychosocial well-being of offspring created as a result of third-party reproduction and assisted reproduction, and in treatment denial decisions. In short, infertility counselling, whether provided by a psychiatrist or other mental health professional, involves the treatment and care of various patients, not simply while they are undergoing infertility treatment but also with their long-term emotional well-being, that of their children, and that of the reproductive helpers who may assist them in achieving biologic or reproductive parenthood.

RECOMMENDED READING

1. Burns LH. Psychiatric aspects of infertility and infertility treatments. Psychiatr Clin North Am 2007;30(4):689–716.
2. De Berardis D, Mazza M, Marini S, Del Nibletto L, Serroni N, Pino MC, Valchera A, Ortolani C, Ciarrocchi F, Martinotti G, Di Giannantonio M. Psychopathology, emotional aspects and psychological counselling in infertility: A review. Clin Ter 2014;165(3):163–9.
3. Leader A, Taylor PJ, Daniluk J. Infertility: Clinical and psychological aspects. Psychiatr Ann 1984;14(6):461–7.
4. Noorbala AA, Ramezanzadeh F, Abedinia N, Naghizadeh MM. Psychiatric disorders among infertile and fertile women. Soc Psych Psychiatr Epidemiol 2009;44(7):587–91.

Psychosocial Aspects of Surrogacy

Hrishikesh Pai, Avinash De Sousa, Rishma Dhillon Pai

INTRODUCTION

- Infertility for any couple is often a subject of shame, ridicule, guilt and stigma in Indian society. Members of society expect Indian couples to complete their reproductive functions and bear children which shall be the requisite to complete the marital function.
- Today in the modern medicine era, this has dwindled and many means of artificial reproductive techniques can be embraced by these couples. Of this, surrogacy is the most controversial and unique method of artificial reproduction. Surrogacy involves another woman, who is a third party apart from the couple in marriage who helps an infertile couple by bearing the child in her womb.
- The womb, child-bearing and pregnancy have their own psychological ramifications for a woman as this often makes up important epochs of her womanhood. The same womanhood when made to depend on another womb, especially depriving a mother of the joys of pregnancy and child-bearing has intense psychosocial diversions.

BASIC CONCEPTS

- When the intended host is inseminated with the semen of the husband of the **'commissioning couple'**, the procedure is known as **'Traditional surrogacy'**, or **'partial surrogacy'**. The resulting child is genetically related to the host. This is illegal and no longer done in India. When the sperm and oocytes of the **'genetic couple'**, or **'commissioning couple'** are used and IVF is carried out on them and the resulting embryos are transferred to the host, this is known as **'gestational surrogacy'**, or **'IVF surrogacy'**.
- **'IVF surrogacy'** has become an accepted treatment option for women in certain countries with these unique circumstances. The surrogate mother is genetically unrelated to the fetus in this arrangement.
- Assisted reproductive technology has enabled both partners in a relationship to use their own gametes to create their own genetic embryos and for these embryos to be transferred to a surrogate host. Women with absent uterus, diseased uterus, with recurrent abortions, recurrent IVF failures and with medical disorders in which pregnancy is contraindicated are able to have her own genetic child through surrogacy.
- "Surrogacy" means an arrangement in which a woman agrees to a pregnancy, achieved through assisted reproductive technology, in which neither of the gametes

belong to her or her husband, with the intention to carry it and handover the child to the person or persons for whom she is acting as a surrogate.

- "Surrogate mother" is the one who agrees to have an embryo generated from the sperm of a man who is not her husband and the oocyte of another woman, implanted in her to carry the pregnancy to viability and deliver the child to the couple/individual that had asked for surrogacy.

GENERAL PSYCHOSOCIAL ISSUES IN SURROGACY

- Until recently surrogacy was rare but with an increase in infertility rates in couples, there has been an increase in couples opting for surrogacy. Surrogacy has in some quarters been commercialized and this had let it become a groundswell of interest and controversy. Surrogacy has faced opposition from many religious and cleric groups who feel that the basic tenets of many a religion have been challenged and violated by surrogacy as a procedure.
- Surrogacy has its share of controversy from a feminist perspective as well. Many feminist rights advocates feel that surrogacy delegitimizes the relationship between a child and mother and leads to a belittling of motherhood and gender roles in women. Many regard it as a form of baby selling which is ridiculing the child-bearing capacity of a woman. Thus, there are various ethical, moral, legal and psychological issues that besiege surrogacy.
- In Indian society, women into surrogacy are thought of as womb sellers and the couple hiring them as womb hirers leading to a gross stigmatization of surrogacy in the first place. The presence of more than two members in the procreation of a child as per Indian society rattles the very pillar a couple whose unison is aimed at a child which will then be labelled as a product of their love.
- The fact that they hire another person to help them get this product fuzzes their relationship and the sanctity of marriage as many traditional Indian groups would agree. In fact, surrogacy is more complex than abortion itself. It is funny that while in many cultural pockets, people do not mind giving up a female child for adoption or engage in female infanticide, they do not feel it leading to a murder of feminism, while surrogacy that in fact gives birth to a new life, actually does.

Psychosocial Issues in a Couple Opting for Surrogacy

- One needs studies that evaluate the psychological mindset of couples that opt for surrogacy as an option in India. These are usually couples from the higher socio-economic strata because surrogacy is not a cheap option in India.
- Studies are needed to evaluate the personality characteristics as well as psychopathology in couples that opt for surrogacy. Usually, these are couples where infertility is a problem and research has seen that infertility is often intertwined with physical, social and psychological factors. The effects of surrogacy on the marital relationship in the long run need evaluation and the dynamics of a third party in the creation of a child needs study.
- Whether the surrogate mother when in regular contact with the commissioning couple affects the couple's attachment and internal dynamics needs a detailed psychological study but consent for the same may be tough to obtain.

Psychosocial Issues in Surrogate Mothers

- One also needs to study the reasons for women entering into surrogacy. Studies done in the past involve reasons ranging from financial payment to a joy obtained by helping someone give birth to a child or procreating a life in general.
- Some studies note an altruistic perspective seen in surrogate mothers who feel a boost to their self-esteem and personal growth when they allow a life in their womb and at the end of 9 months bring joy to the couple. Many surrogate mothers have reported having undergone an abortion in the past as well report having given up a child for adoption and thus understand the plight of a couple that do not have children.
- Surrogates themselves believe surrogacy takes a special type of person. Somehow, they say, they 'know' if they can do a genetic surrogacy that is if they can or cannot relinquish a baby that is genetically theirs. Some surrogates are very young and may not understand the consequences and regret their decisions later at the time of relinquishment or even later in life, when it is too late to do anything about it.

ISSUES RELATED TO ANONYMITY, CONTACT AND GIVING UP THE BABY

- Many surrogates in the UK unequivocally said they believed the commissioning mothers should disclose the arrangement to their surrogate child/children. Where 'closed' arrangements have been used, regrets have been reported. Disclosure can have 'barbaric' consequences for the surrogate and can be as dramatically perceived by the child once he/she finds out.
- Similar concerns have been expressed concerning an anonymous arrangement as well. In India, most surrogacy arrangements are anonymous and disclosure would have similar consequences as in any other nation. Conceiving, carrying and delivering a baby is the start of a process of care and commitment to nurture the baby through childhood and into adulthood. This is culturally expected and more so in India.
- Having a social termination of pregnancy or giving a child up for adoption are controversies to the accepted norm, and for surrogacy, where the surrogate conceives only to give the baby up following delivery, the process is even more unconventional. Theoretically, women are known to develop varying degrees of attachment to their baby during pregnancy and this is carried over to the baby following birth.
- Surrogate mothers tend to be between 25 and 35 years, and most believe they have completed their own family. Research, which has looked at attachment, has found that surrogate mothers are less attached to the baby and less attached to the baby following delivery.
- Consequently, surrogate mothers do not allow themselves to be attached to the baby or infant following delivery. The practice of handling the baby over to the commissioning couples straight after birth also reinforces the advice. The surrogate agencies assist surrogates in reconciling their own maternal thoughts and feelings, by cognitively restructuring these feelings to match their behaviours' (relinquishment of the baby).
- A few surrogates report feeling exploited and many surrogates involve their own family in the surrogate process. In addition, surrogate mothers expected their commissioning parents to be open about the child's origins, as they themselves had

told all their own children about the surrogate baby being part of the intended couple's family—not their own. As a result of this, most surrogate mothers expected some contact between them to continue following relinquishment of the baby, so that they maintained their new friendships and their children could still see the surrogate child. It was argued that this made it easier for their own children to understand what is involved and who the couples are who will have their mother's 'tummy baby'.

- Unfortunately, in some cases, this contact ceased unexpectedly after the legal proceedings had been completed. It is seen as a betrayal when the intended couple with the surrogate baby disappears from the surrogate and her children's lives. The long-term care and support for surrogate mothers is not always considered by intended couples, once they remove themselves from the surrogates' life. Further longitudinal research on surrogate mothers is needed, and this should also address the well-being of the surrogate's own children.

PSYCHOLOGICAL ISSUES IN COMMISSIONING MOTHERS

- Surrogacy offers a unique option for infertile mothers. It differs from adoption because it allows for a full or partial genetic link with the child and differs from adoption because a pregnancy is not possible. Other reasons were because they would have a full or partial genetic link with the child or because IVF or adoption failed.

- A few psychological studies have been carried out on intended mothers, and even less is available on the fathers. In general, surrogacy was largely initiated through information from the media and was based on gut feelings in the matching process and trust (the surrogate trusting the commissioning couple to pay the fee; the commissioning couple trusting the surrogate to care for the baby *in utero* and relinquish it upon delivery).

- Another important observation made in studies of commissioning mothers is that intended mothers were not inclined to attempt to justify their unusual choice. An explanation for the few infertile women opting for surrogacy is the contributing biological force. Accounts of commissioning mothers show that most intend to tell their child from an early age how they were conceived and carried. American guidelines tend to encourage openness about origins to the child (even in some closed programmes), but the guidelines do not specify how and when the optimum time to tell the child is.

- Openness about conception, gestation and genetic origins has practical reasons too, particularly in the UK, where many surrogate and recipient couples develop a strong bond or friendship, as physical and emotional changes are relevant to both parties. Many couples also experience tremendous ups and downs, e.g. the joy when the result of a pregnancy test is positive and the experience of birth is shared, or if a pregnancy has not been established or results in a miscarriage both parties suffer together under these difficult conditions.

- They, therefore, get to know each other intimately for the duration of at least a year and most intend to keep in contact well after the arrangement has terminated. It is difficult to state whether similar findings may be found and reciprocated in Indian populations.

PSYCHOLOGICAL ISSUES IN SURROGATE OFFSPRING

There is a paucity of information on surrogate offspring, even though there are now at least several hundred children born as a result of surrogate arrangements. This figure is likely to be larger, because not all surrogate and commissioning couples feedback to the agencies, if they successfully completed these arrangements, and some are known to take place outside of any involvement of organizations, making accurate documentation impossible.

UNDECIDED PSYCHOSOCIAL ISSUES IN SURROGACY

- Surrogacy arrangements may be of two types—commercial and altruistic. Almost no legislation has attempted to define the two. Generally, commercial surrogacy arrangements are those involving payments made to surrogate, which are over and above the necessary medical expenses. This is common when the surrogate is unknown to the commissioning couple. Altruistic arrangements are associated with no or only minimum payments for the necessary medical expenses. This is more commonly arranged between close relatives and friends of the commissioning parents. However, the task of clearly differentiating the two arrangements has always been troublesome.
- In India, it has been realized that though surrogacy arrangements are a viable option for infertile couples, it involves strong human emotions. This highly emotional issue has been tactfully dealt with while attempting to decide on whom, the parental rights should be conferred, so that the welfare of the child is not undermined. The national guidelines have elaborately laid down the suggested law. It does not consider the surrogate to be the legal mother under any circumstances. It explains that in cases where the surrogate is bearing a child with whom she has no genetic relation, the birth certificate shall have the name of the genetic parent.
- It is important to consider whether payments are the only factor which induces a surrogate to undertake risks which at times could run contrary to her best interests. Some believe that only commercial arrangements are exploitative by nature, while altruistic arrangements are considerably less abusive. While trying to gauge the level of exploitation in each type of arrangement, it is necessary, to take into account both economical and emotional exploitations, in one's deliberations.

RECOMMENDED READING

1. Ber R. Ethical issues in gestational surrogacy. Theoret Med Bioethics 2000;21(2):153–69.
2. Ciccarelli JC, Beckman LJ. Navigating rough waters: An overview of psychological aspects of surrogacy. J Soc Issues 2005;61(1):21–43.
3. Edelmann RJ. Surrogacy: The psychological issues. J Reprod Infant Psychol 2004;22(2):123–36.
4. Kumar P, Inder D, Sharma N. Surrogacy and women's right to health in India: Issues and perspective. Indian J Pub Health 2013;57(2):65–9.
5. Teman E. The social construction of surrogacy research: An anthropological critique of the psychosocial scholarship on surrogate motherhood. Soc Sci Med 2008;67(7):1104–12.

Section

IV

Psychological Issues in Gynaecology

CHAPTER

9

Ashwini Bhalerao Gandhi, Komal Chavan, Sneha Venkateswaran

Psychological Issues in Adolescence

WHO defines 'adolescents' as individuals in the age group of 10–19 years. Individuals in the age group 15–24 years are referred to as 'youth', while those in the age group 10–24 years are called 'young people'. Adolescents exist in a variety of circumstances and have special needs. This is the period of transition from being a child to being an adult. It involves various physical, psychological, sexual and social developmental changes. Although this is a time for growth and development of an individual in many aspects, it also poses risks to their health and wellbeing.

This chapter highlights the psychological issues in adolescents in various clinical scenarios.

GENERAL PRINCIPLES

An adolescent girl may have a lot of fear and anxiety during a gynaecological examination. It is necessary to adopt a calm, gentle, sensitive and patient approach to win her and her attendant's confidence. Sometimes, it may be necessary to interview the girl alone without her parents' interference and assure her confidentiality for the information shared. It is important to document all the problems that the girl is going through without any bias or prejudice and keeping in mind her mental and psychological status. Even in the phase of normal pubertal development, there are abundant emotional and psychological changes. There may be a sense of crisis in the search for identity and sexual development. There may be psychological stress, turmoil or even depressive psychosis in the growing child. Rising gonadal steroid levels are responsible for these changes.

PRECOCIOUS PUBERTY

Sexual precocity is defined as appearance of any of the secondary sexual characters at an age which is less than 2 standard deviations below the mean for that population. It may be of the True (central) type or Pseudo (peripheral) type. In such cases, psychological support is needed for both children and their parents. The children need to be protected from sexual assault. Patient and parent education and group counselling therapies are of help. Cases of bullying in school may lead to poor school performance and depressive symptoms. Knowing all these features as a group and addressing them together along with medical treatment of the condition (with GnRH analogues) help in optimum treatment of precocious puberty.

DELAYED PUBERTY

This is defined as the lack of physical manifestations of sexual maturation in boys and girls at an age that is 2 standard deviations above the mean age of puberty for that population. The most common psychological problem that these children experience is peer pressure of being shorter and less 'developed' than their colleagues. The most common cause of delayed puberty is physiological delay. Detailed history should be sought regarding the age of onset of puberty in the mother and sisters of the child. School health education classes are essential to avoid the psychological trauma that children face on a daily basis leading to poor school performance.

Apart from these, the gynaecologist should be aware and consider the possibility of disorders of sex development (intersex) in children who develop abnormal virilization/feminization during puberty. Proper medical or surgical management must be instituted in these cases.

MENSTRUAL DYSFUNCTION

Although some degree of dysfunctional uterine bleeding (DUB) in puberty is common and due to anovulation, some girls may go through a prolonged anovulatory phase leading to heavy, prolonged and irregular cycles. This can lead to significant psychological distress among girls and their parents due to unpredictable bleeding days and disturbance in activities of daily living. Apart from medical management of DUB and supportive management with haematinics, psychological support in the form of education, counselling, behaviour therapy is necessary for the management of menstrual dysfunction in puberty. Diet, exercise and counselling therapy is also needed for the management of premenstrual syndrome (PMS) and premenstrual dysphonic disorder (PMDD).

TEENAGE PREGNANCY

Media, peer pressure, family structure and values have an influence on teenage sexuality. Accurate knowledge of contraceptive practices and reproductive biology is poor among common people. Also, the rising incidence of sexual assault in adolescent girls may even lead to unwanted pregnancies among them. Besides having adverse implications on the health of the teen mother, it also limits her education and career opportunities. Uneducated women may be prevented from using family planning services. Girls from broken families often become sexually involved in an attempt to find a kind of caring which is lacking in their homes. Very few of these young girls have had sex education at home or in their schools. Indeed, sex education is the single most important measure to ensure reduction in teenage pregnancies and encourage safe sex practices. Prevention of dangerous practices and sensitive management of adolescent sexuality ensure a healthy womanhood.

APPROACHES FOR PSYCHOTHERAPY IN ADOLESCENTS

There are four recognized methods of psychotherapy in adolescents:
1. **Family therapy:** It helps families find positive and productive ways to communicate. Some therapy sessions may involve the parents only or the children only, or both together. It aims to bring about workable solutions for everyone involved.

2. **Group therapy:** Combining patients or groups of them may help in giving comfort to some individuals when they learn that there are others facing the same kind of problems. These group sessions also turn out to be less expensive.
3. **Cognitive behaviour therapy (CBT):** In this, the therapist helps the child understand how his mood can directly affect his behaviour. This helps individuals cope with anxiety, depression and post-traumatic stress disorder.
4. **Play therapy:** Usually reserved for younger children, it uses the observation of the way a child plays for the therapist to piece together the child's emotional life. Then the therapist can use a combination of conversations and activities to help the child productively process his or her emotions, thoughts and behaviours.

RECOMMENDED READING

1. Cheng S, Chan ACM.The multidimensional scale of perceived social support: Dimensionality and age and gender differences in adolescents. Personality and Individual Differences, 2004; 37:1359–69.
2. Rutter M, Graham P, Chadwick O F D et al. Adolescent Turmoil, fact or fiction? Child Psychol Psychiatry 1976;17:35–36.

Premenstrual Syndrome

Ashwini Bhalerao Gandhi, Avinash De Sousa, Komal Chavan

Premenstrual syndrome (PMS) is also sometimes known as premenstrual tension (PMT). One in three women suffers discomforting symptoms in the days before their period. For one in 20, the symptoms are bad enough to more seriously affect their lives.

SYMPTOMS

There are more than 100 recognized symptoms linked to PMS, but most women only experience a handful of them. Symptoms can be both psychological (mental) and physical.

The most common are:

1. **Psychological PMS symptoms**
   - Irritability and mood swings
   - Loss of confidence
   - Feeling angry
   - Feeling upset and emotional
   - Depressed mood
   - Tearfulness
   - Anxiety
   - Tiredness
   - Poor concentration
   - Restlessness
2. **Physical PMS symptoms**
   - Weight gain
   - Abdominal bloating
   - Tender and lumpy breasts
   - Swollen ankles
   - Headaches
   - Backaches
   - Skin changes and acne
   - Upset stomach
   - Insomnia
   - Tiredness

- Joint aches
- Dizziness

3. **Behavioural PMS symptoms**
    - Food cravings and overeating
    - Loss of interest in sex

The International Society for Premenstrual Disorders (ISPMD) defined precise criteria for diagnosing premenstrual disorders (PMD), and divided PMS into core and variant. In all PMD, symptoms should cause impairment of daily activities at work, social activities and interpersonal relationships.

Core (or typical) PMD is associated with spontaneous ovulatory menstrual cycles and may be subdivided into predominantly physical symptoms, predominantly psychological or mixed. Women whose symptoms are predominantly psychological or mixed may also fulfil the criteria for premenstrual dysphoric disorder.

Variants of PMD encompass more complex features, divided into the four following categories:

1. Premenstrual exacerbation of an underlying condition
2. PMS in the absence of menstruation
3. Progestogen-induced PMS
4. PMS with anovulatory ovarian activity.

CAUSES OF PMS

- Too much salty food can contribute to fluid retention and bloating.
- Fizzy drinks and alcohol can reduce your energy levels and disrupt mood.
- Low levels of vitamins and minerals may also worsen PMS symptoms.

Exactly what causes premenstrual syndrome is unknown, but several factors may contribute to the condition:

- Signs and symptoms of premenstrual syndrome change with hormonal fluctuations and disappear with pregnancy and menopause.
- Fluctuations of serotonin, a brain chemical (neurotransmitter) that is thought to play a crucial role in mood states, could trigger PMS symptoms. Insufficient amounts of serotonin may contribute to premenstrual depression, as well as to fatigue, food cravings and sleep problems.
- Some women with severe premenstrual syndrome have undiagnosed depression, though depression alone does not cause all of the symptoms.

Since mood and behavioural symptoms are key features of PMS, underlying mechanisms must involve the brain. Indeed, sex steroids easily pass the blood–brain barrier, and sex steroid receptors are abundant in many brain regions that regulate emotions and behaviour, including the amygdala and the hypothalamus.

The brain neurotransmitter serotonin is implicated in the regulation of mood and behaviour, partly because of observations made in preclinical studies, and partly because of the antidepressant and anxiety-reducing effects exerted by serotonin-facilitating drugs in human beings. This notion has also gained support from genetic studies and from brain imaging experiments.

DIAGNOSIS

There is no laboratory test that can diagnose PMS, although blood and urine tests can rule out other causes. The condition is recognized by noting the type of symptoms and when they occur in relation to the period. Keeping a diary for a few months will help you to recognize PMS symptoms and when to expect them, and will also help with diagnosis.

Some symptoms of PMS are shared by other conditions such as depression, anxiety, menopause, chronic fatigue syndrome (CFS), irritable bowel syndrome (IBS) and thyroid gland problems. A few women find that their symptoms are severe enough to stop them living their normal life due to more intense PMS, called premenstrual dysphoric disorder.

TREATMENT OF PMS

- Understanding the condition is the first step. For most women, the symptoms are a mild inconvenience which they can deal with themselves.
- Keep a diary to help predict when PMS symptoms are due. Try to manage stress levels around that time, e.g. rearrange potentially difficult meetings, avoid having guests to stay, arrange extra childcare, etc.
- Make sure you get enough sleep, try to get 8 hours every night.
- Stop smoking.
- Talk about it to family and friends so they can understand how you are feeling.
- If bloating is a problem, wear loose, comfortable clothing with an elasticated waist band and a more supportive bra.
- Relaxation and gentle exercise are beneficial.
- Eating the right foods should lessen the symptoms of PMS.
- Generally, you should try to consume less junk food, fat, sugar, salt, caffeine and alcohol, and eat more starch, fibre, vegetables and fruit. It also helps to eat small meals regularly.

A number of treatments are available. Some may be more effective than others. Treatments may take several months to work fully and may not cure symptoms completely but symptoms often become less frequent or easier with treatment. The treatment of PMS is a fast-growing area of research.

Hormone Treatments

- **Combined oral contraceptive pill:** Thought to alleviate PMS by stopping ovulation and reducing hormonal fluctuations. However, in some women, the hormones in the pill cause PMS. If symptoms return in the pill-free interval, then the pill can be taken continuously and a seven-day breaks only taken, if breakthrough bleeding occurs.
- **Oestrogen patches and implants:** There is scientific evidence that extra oestrogen given this way can relieve PMS symptoms by suppressing ovulation and reducing hormonal fluctuations.
- **Mirena intrauterine system (IUS):** This is a contraceptive coil which releases a small dose of a progestogen. Some women say it improves PMS, as well as reducing the heaviness and duration of their period.

- Other powerful medicines called luteinizing hormone-releasing hormone (LHRH) analogues are available which temporarily switch off the ovaries. They are reserved for severe cases of PMS.
- Gonadotrophin-releasing hormone analogues are drugs that prevent ovulation and should only be used for the treatment of severe PMS. Although thesework well, menopausal sideeffects commonly occur which limit their usefulness in treating PMS.

Non-Hormonal Treatments

- **Selective serotonin re-uptake inhibitors (SSRIs):** An SSRI medicine is commonly prescribed to treat more severe PMS. These medicines were first developed to treat depression. However, they have also been found to ease the symptoms of PMS, even if one is not depressed. They work by increasing the level of serotonin in the brain. These have been shown to relieve the symptoms of tiredness, low mood, food cravings and sleep problems. They do have side effects which sometimes outweigh their usefulness for PMS sufferers but there are various brands. Research suggests that taking an SSRI for just half of the menstrual cycle (the second half of the monthly cycle) is as effective as taking an SSRI all of the time.
- **Diuretics (water tablets)** such as spironolactone may help relieve premenstrual bloating, breast tenderness, and weight gain.
- **Cognitive-behaviour therapy (CBT):** This is a psychological treatment, during which ways to find more adaptive ways of coping with premenstrual symptoms are explored. This has been shown to be effective for some women.
- A hysterectomy with removal of both ovaries to prevent ovulation may be necessary for a few women who suffer from severe PMS. Removing the uterus without the ovaries may not improve the symptoms as there will still be fluctuations in the hormonal cycle. This is a drastic treatment and will only be undertaken in severe cases and if all other treatments have been unsuccessful.

Non-Prescription Treatments

- Over the counter pain relievers (such as ibuprofen and paracetamol) can help ease symptoms such as cramps, headaches, backaches and breast tenderness.
- Although there is little scientific evidence, many women have found significant relief from some PMS symptoms by using complementary or alternative therapies.
- St John's Wort: This is a herbal remedy shown to alleviate mild to moderate depression which can bepurchased from pharmacies. There is limited evidenceto show it is effective in treating PMS. It may interfere with the efficacy of the combined contraceptive pill.
- Evening primrose oil (EPO) is a source of gamma linoleic acid and is helpful in alleviating premenstrual breast pain in some women.
- Black cohosh, wild yam root, agnus castus(chaste berry) and dong quai have also been reported to help with PMS symptoms but there is only limited evidence to support this.

Vitamins and Minerals

- Some women with PMS have lower magnesium levels, although further research is needed.

- Calcium and vitamin D taken together may help with premenstrual pain and migraine.
- Vitamin B$_6$, also known as pyridoxine. For some women, it helps with the symptoms of mood swings and irritability. It can be taken everyday or just for two weeks before a period. Be careful not to exceed the maximum daily dose.
- Folic acid to help alleviate fatigue and depression.
- Natural diuretics are available over the counter to help with swelling and bloating.

At the outset, it is important to establish a precise diagnosis and not rely on the patient's own diagnosis. It is mandatory to separate PMS/PMDD from other diagnoses, particularly depression and anxiety disorders, premenstrual exacerbation of another disorder, or mild physiological symptoms requiring no more than reassurance; preferably this assessment should be done by the general practitioner before referral to a gynaecologist or a psychiatrist.

Diagnosis is best achieved through daily rating symptoms over at least one menstrual cycle; clinicians can ask patients to choose their worst symptoms and chart the severity daily, or can select a validated scale such as the Daily Record of Severity of Problems. The disappearance of symptoms after menstruation is the key to diagnosis.

PMS does not seem to be due to abnormal concentrations of sex steroids, but the symptoms are triggered by fluctuations of such hormones, the difference between patients and controls probably being that patients are more sensitive to such fluctuations. With respect to brain function, the transmitters serotonin and GABA have been implicated in the underlying mechanism.

Treatments inhibiting ovulation, such as GnRH analogues, oestrogen and certain new oral contraceptives effectively reduce the symptoms, as do treatment with SRIs, which by some institutions are regarded as first-line agents in severely affected patients.

RECOMMENDED READING

1. Bancroft J, Bäckström T. Premenstrual syndrome. Clin Endocrinol 1985;22(3):313–36.
2. Braverman PK. Premenstrual syndrome and premenstrual dysphoric disorder. J Pediatr Adolesc Gynecol 2007;20(1):3–12.
3. Dickerson LM, Mazyck PJ, Hunter MH. Premenstrual syndrome. Am Fam Physician 2003;67(8): 1743–52.
4. Rapkin A. A review of treatment of premenstrual syndrome and premenstrual dysphoric disorder. Psychoneuroendocrinology 2003;28:39–53.
5. Yonkers KA, O'Brien PS, Eriksson E. Premenstrual syndrome. Lancet 2008;371(9619):1200–10.

Psychiatric Side Effects of Hormones and Oral Contraceptive Pills

Avinash De Sousa, Komal Chavan, Priyanka Sonawane

- Although research on hormonal contraceptive side effects has been vastly under reported in recent times, an awareness of the adverse effects is important for every patient and physician who encounters hormonal contraceptive users. As with any medication, hormonal contraceptives have side effects, some of which can even be deadly.
- Dr. CR Kay and the Royal College of General Practitioners were one of the first groups to study the pill and its associated side effects. A cohort of approximately 46,000 women was followed for 25 years.
- Six years into the study the first major interim report was published which showed several significant correlations among users. Among those include: A 30% relative increase in depression, a fourfold decrease in libido, an increase in divorce.
- Twenty-five years after the study's inception, newer associations dealing with physical side effects emerged; however, the potential psychological impact of this class of drugs still remained exemplified by their association with all violent and accidental causes of death. It is interesting to note that in the first 10 years of oral contraceptive pill (OCP) use, there was a significant excess of mortality from all causes of death.
- An interesting observation, however, is made in the interim report concerning the fact that neurotic depression did not vary with the hormonal dose given. The authors speculate a possible non-pharmacological effect as the cause.
- It is interesting to note one of the few significant differences is that OCP users had four times as many suicide attempts compared with diaphragm users. And suicides among ages 50–64. Another study also of older women on hormone replacement therapy (the British HRT Study) likewise revealed a statistically increased number of deaths from suicide.
- Although these side effects are considered by some to be too small to discourage their use given the benefit of such high contraceptive efficacy, many users would disagree.
- During the early years of hormonal contraceptive use, it was surprising to somehow the side effects could so lead to a very significant discontinuation rate. Some of the aforementioned studies, as well as other recent studies, reveal substantial rates of discontinuation secondary to experiencing side effects. It appears that even with the advent of newer more "user friendly" hormonal preparations, there has been little change in the discontinuation rate and overall satisfaction.

- The importance of the emotional side effects of hormonal contraception is there. Ever since the interim results of the first major cohort studies were released, more attention has been focused on the emotional and behavioural side effects of hormonal contraceptives. In the late 1960s, it was formally noted that there was a prevalence of two life-disturbing behavioural side effects of the hormonal preparations: Depression and decreased libido.
- While relatively few will suffer the consequences of the contraceptive's emotional side effects to the extreme of committing suicide, many have sympathized with those of depression, anxiety, and even apparent subsequent sexual dysfunction which is commonly cited in the literature.
- Rosemarie Lincoln in writing on the loss of libido points to the following effects as leading many times to the loss of sexual interest in a relationship: Depression, grief, the need for self-punishment or control, unconscious anger.
- Likewise, Bozeman and Beck demonstrated that anger reduces men's sexual desire and penile tumescence. Not only does emotional pathology seem to pose a problem in itself to hormonal contraceptive users, but it also seems to lead to further psychosocial and relational problems.
- For example, the theory that progesterone is responsible for decreased sexual interest, as is also observed in primates, seems to be refuted by observations that some women who discontinue such contraceptives become less interested in sex than others.

Male	Female
In utero • Testosterone and its aromatization to estrogen cause masculinization of the fetal brain	**In utero** • Absence of androgen production and estrogen-binding activity of alpha-fetoprotein cause feminization of the fetal brain
Adolescence • More between-network connectivity • Larger grey matter volume • Lower grey matter density	**Adolescence** • More within-network connectivity • Less grey matter volume • Higher grey matter density
Adulthood • More total brain volume • More grey matter volume • More white matter volume • More cerebrospinal fluid volume • Higher proportion of white matter • Larger volume of the central subdivision of the bed nucleus stria terminalis • Better visuospatial and mathematical ability • Weaker right-hand preference	**Adulthood** • Less total brain volume • Less grey matter volume • Less white matter volume • Less cerebrospinal fluid volume • Higher proportion of grey matter • Thicker cortex • Higher global cerebral blood flow • Better perceptual speed and fine manual dexterity • Stronger right-hand preference

Fig. 11.1: Effects of hormones on the developing brain

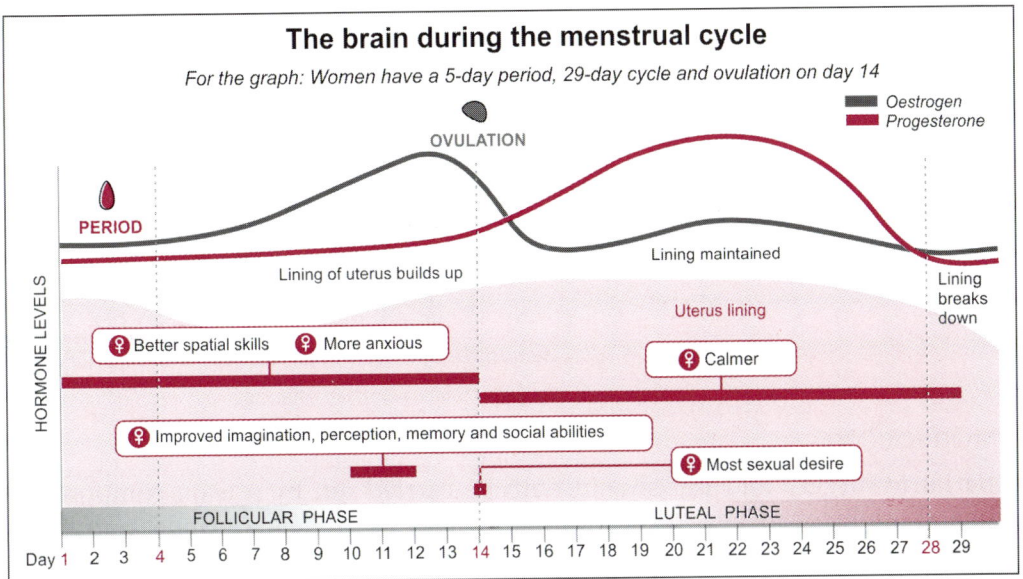

Fig. 11.2: The effect of the menstrual cycle on the brain

As research continues, new tools are continually being developed to further aid in identifying cause and effect relationships from correlatives and associations. The primary study designs in the above studied literature have been limited to large cohorts, small RCTs using placebo and non-users, cross-sectional analyses, and the use of standardized psychological instruments. Given the significant emotional disturbances associated with the intentional administration of what a woman thinks is a contraceptive is enough to warrant further study. If this association is accurate, then one would have to consider the possibility that contraceptive behaviour itself has inherent detrimental side effects. Now is the time for a definitive breakthrough in characterizing this relationship. There is now solid research identifying a new effective way to postpone pregnancy called natural family planning (NFP). By definition, it would technically not fall into the category of contraception and would seem to not have such associated emotional side effects, if the hypothesis proposed is true. There are also very well validated psychological instruments available which would allow research to uncover accurate associations of emotional disturbances in comparison to a normal population control group (Figs 11.1 and 11.2).

Psychological Aspects of Bariatric Surgery and Obesity in Women

Avinash De Sousa, Niranjan Chavan, Priyanka Sonawane

INTRODUCTION

- Bariatric surgery and BIB should both be carried out by a team composed of multidisciplinary members. The ideal clinical practice guideline includes nutritional, metabolic, and non-surgical support before and after bariatric surgery. The presurgical assessment performed by the psychiatrists involves the candidates' ability to understand the surgical procedure, make a responsible decision, and adhere to postsurgical management.
- As a result, bariatric surgery candidates with psychiatric symptoms or a psychiatric diagnosis may have a higher risk of dropout prior to surgery. The decision to turn down a bariatric surgery candidate remains controversial. Psychopathology of the candidate as a contraindication to bariatric surgery can be absolute or relative, depending on the adhesiveness of the multidisciplinary team.
- More devoted involvement from mental health providers may improve the care quality and safety of bariatric surgery patients.

PSYCHIATRIC PROBLEMS IN THOSE UNDERGOING BARIATRIC SURGERY

- The high prevalence of psychiatric disorders in surgery candidates is gaining more attention than before. Studies from several countries show that around 40% of all bariatric surgery patients have at least one psychiatric diagnosis.
- Depressive disorders (dysthymic disorder and major depressive disorder), anxiety disorders (e.g. generalized anxiety disorder), and eating disorders (i.e. binge eating disorder) are the three commonest psychiatric diagnoses.
- Identification of these disorders improves the quality of perioperative management and helps predict the weight loss outcome after bariatric surgery. For example, a lifetime history of mood disorder implies poor weight loss.
- Eating pattern is also important in presurgical assessment. An absence of binge-eating behaviour is associated with a favourable weight loss result after surgery. Bariatric surgery candidates may be especially prone to eating-related disorders, internalized weight bias, and body shame.
- Substance use disorder like alcohol abuse is another critical issue, as bariatric surgery candidates may have a greater lifetime risk of alcohol use disorders and a greater propensity to alcohol intoxication after bariatric surgery.

- Apart from this, personality factors also are associated with mood symptoms and eating behaviours among bariatric surgery candidates. Neurotic personality traits are associated with more concerns about body figure, binge-eating driven by stress, more depression and anxiety, and more negative coping reactions.
- Bariatric surgery candidates are also likely to have had previous suicide attempts. Patients with a positive suicide history may have a greater BMI. One of the possible explanations for the high suicide risk among bariatric surgery candidates is stigma. Overweight-related stigma may make an individual more vulnerable to social isolation, and hence is associated with suicidal ideation and behaviour.
- Sexual abuse history is associated with poorer weight loss outcomes following bariatric treatment. Alcohol addiction, psychiatric comorbidities, and low-income status are highly associated with sexual abuse. A physical abuse history, suicidal ideation, and psychiatric symptoms also are associated with sexual abuse or physical attack status in bariatric surgery patients.

Psychological Management

- Presurgical pharmaceutical and non-pharmaceutical management is suggested for bariatric surgery candidates in need of stabilizing the mental status.
- Cognitive-behavioural therapy (CBT) is effective in treating psychopathology regardless of the presence of binge-eating disorder or degree of obesity. In a study of 3-month CBT programme with twelve 2-h sessions before bariatric surgery, candidates' self-esteem, depression, and eating disorders were much improved especially in those with binge eating disorder.
- After bariatric surgery, mental health professionals need to regularly monitor the progress of weight loss and the occurrence or worsening of psychiatric symptoms. Postsurgical assessment and systematic follow-up are necessary to guarantee optimal weight loss and weight regain prevention.
- The presence of depressive disorders after bariatric surgery may predict attenuated weight loss after treatment.
- More recent studies point out the tendency of improved cognitive function after bariatric surgery. Memory improvement in bariatric surgery patients is noted after 12 months. Post-surgery cognitive function is important because it may predict future weight loss. Better cognition helps weight loss as cognitive function is associated with adherence to the post-surgical guidelines dealing with diet, exercise, and other lifestyle changes.
- Suicide attempts and risk of completed suicide among bariatric surgery patients deserve much attention in the follow-up period. There seems to be a positive association between obesity and suicide, but some studies do not favour this association. Unlike other psychopathologies that improve after bariatric surgery, suicide risk remains high and warrants long-term supervision.
- Psychotherapy such as behavioural-motivational nutritional education or behavioural psychotherapy may improve depressive symptoms after bariatric surgery. This improvement in depression can then lead to more ideal weight loss. Obese patients receiving weight management services can achieve better psychosocial health.

- Like the adult population, obese adolescents also have high rates of psychopathology. However, the youth population may have different causes. Childhood experience of parental loss is associated with metabolic syndrome. After bariatric surgery, adolescents may experience marked improvement in depressive symptoms, binge-eating, and quality of life. Interfamilial conflict, on the other hand, may hamper weight loss after surgery among youth. School problems and cognitive impairment are found to be associated with increased BMI among younger bariatric candidates. Therefore, improving academic support and deficiencies in educational systems for obese students is necessary to make the assessment and intervention complete.
- The role of sex in obesity and bariatric surgery is another unsolved issue. One study found no significant difference in weight loss between men and women after bariatric surgery. Another study indicated that men and women differ significantly in terms of suspected psychosurgical risk factors like depression and anxiety. Assessments of bariatric surgery candidates should recognize that men and women have different baseline risk factors, and the reported results should be separated by sex. For example, female bariatric surgery candidates with infertility may be more psychiatrically vulnerable than other bariatric surgery patients. These candidates receive less psychiatric treatment than their counterparts.

PSYCHOLOGICAL PROBLEMS IN FEMALE PATIENTS WITH OBESITY

- Epidemiological studies support positive associations between BMI and mood disorders. There has been found increased odds of mood disorder symptoms including major depression, dysthymia, and manic and hypomanic episodes among obese and extremely obese persons compared with their normal-weight counterparts.
- Obese individuals were 1.5 times more likely than normal-weight individuals to report lifetime or past-year mood disorder; extremely obese persons were twice as likely. Anxiety disorder rates were elevated not only in the obese and extremely obese but also in those who were only moderately overweight.
- Relationships between elevated body weight and affective disorders appear stronger in women than in men. Obesity was associated with mood and anxiety disorders in both men and women. Other studies have found obesity to be related to depression in women but not in men. There is even some evidence that overweight and obesity may be associated with a lower likelihood of attempting or committing suicide among men, although increased BMI is associated with a greater likelihood of suicidal ideation among women.
- Concerns that they will be scrutinized or judged based on weight may contribute to social anxiety in overweight and obese women. In fact, overweight and obese women are at increased risk for social phobia, but BMI is not associated with the likelihood of social phobia among men.
- Mood and anxiety disorders can lead to weight gain by interfering with healthy eating or regular exercise. Eating may have an anxiolytic effect, although overeating in response to stress varies between individuals. Women are more likely than men to eat in response to negative emotions, and women with mood disorders are more likely than men to report increased appetite as a symptom of depression.
- Associations between obesity and mood and anxiety disorders may arise from effects of stress on the hypothalamic-pituitary-adrenal (HPA) axis, which responds to stress

by releasing cortisol and other hormones that modulate sympathetic nervous system activity. Under conditions of chronic stress, HPA axis activity becomes dysregulated, a state that has been implicated in depression and anxiety disorders as well as in obesity.

- Epidemiological studies of relationships between obesity and substance use disorders yield inconsistent findings. Higher rates of lifetime alcohol use disorders among overweight, obese, and extremely obese individuals.
- Significant associations between BMI and illicit drug use disorders have not been identified. However, epidemiological samples include a few persons with drug use disorders because of low population base rates.
- Compulsive overeating and addictions to alcohol and other drugs appear to share common psychological and physiological underpinnings. Intake of food or drugs is reinforcing and activates reward circuits in the brain, causing the release of dopamine.
- Obesity is associated with several personality disorders. Antisocial, avoidant, obsessive-compulsive, paranoid, and schizoid personality disorders are all more prevalent among the obese and extremely obese than in normal-weight persons. In addition, extreme obesity is associated with a greater likelihood of dependent personality disorder. Antisocial personality disorder (ASPD) is significantly associated with BMI among women.
- Obesity has been associated with elevated rates of attention-deficit/hyperactivity disorder (ADHD). Children with ADHD and other disruptive behaviour disorders are heavier than their peers without behavioural disorders and are likely to remain overweight into adulthood. Impulsivity associated with ADHD may thus contribute to overeating and obesity.
- Schizophrenia is not associated with obesity after controlling for other variables. However, treatment with antipsychotic medications particularly olanzapine and clozapine can lead to substantial weight gain in some patients.

RECOMMENDED READING

1. Denmark F, Paludi MA (editors). Psychology of women: Handbook of Issues and Theories. Greenwood Publishing Group; 2007.
2. Fikkan JL, Rothblum ED. Is fat a feminist issue? Exploring the gendered nature of weight bias. Sex Roles 2012;66(9–10):575–92.
3. Hebebrand J, Herpertz-Dahlmann B. Psychological and psychiatric aspects of pediatric obesity. Child Adolesc Psychiatr Clin North Am 2009;18(1):49–65.
4. Sarwer DB, Fabricatore AN, Jones-Corneille LR, Allison KC, Faulcon bridge LN, Wadden TA. Psychological issues following bariatric surgery. Prim Psychiatry 2008;15(8):50–5.
5. Song A, Fernstrom MH. Nutritional and psychological considerations after bariatric surgery. Aesth Surg J 2008;28(2):195–9.

Psychological Aspects of Hysterectomy

Tejasvi Dave, Sushma Sonavane, Komal Chavan, Sneha Venkateswaran

DEFINITION

Hysterectomy is the removal of the uterine corpus with (total hysterectomy) or without the cervix (subtotal or supracervical hysterectomy). It can be done by laparotomy, vaginally, by applying minimally invasive techniques (laparoscopy, robotic surgery) or a combination of two.

Depending on the reason of removal, ovaries and fallopian tubes may also be removed (Table 13.1). After hysterectomy, menstrual cycle will be discontinued and the woman will no longer be able to conceive. Hysterectomy is usually performed as the last option.

EFFECTS

- Hysterectomy causes the oestrogen levels to drop. This results in mood swings, irritability, hot flashes, breasts tenderness, weight gain, fatigue, depressive features and dyspareunia due to dryness in the vagina. Along with changes in the diet, many women opt for hormone replacement therapy.
- Some women feel less interested in sex post-hysterectomy, especially if the ovaries are removed. However, some woman report improved sexual functioning.
- Hysterectomy in the child-bearing years can be extremely distressing for the woman planning a family.
- A lot of women associate womanhood with the reproductive system and feels that it gives them the worth of being a woman. Post-hysterectomy, they feel depressed

Table 13.1: Indications for hysterectomy
• Leiomyoma (fibroids)
• Endometriosis
• Cervical dysplasia
• Menstrual disorders refractory to medical management
• Uterine prolapse
• Endometrial hyperplasia
• Uterine cancer
• Obstetric indications (postpartum haemorrhage, rupture uterus, etc.)

over a loss of fertility. They often report of feeling emptiness and a part of womanhood missing. Occasionally, sense of identity is affected. However, it seldom results in increased anxiety disorders, major depression or other major psychiatric morbidity.

- On the other hand, a lot of women also report improvement in emotional well-being due to alleviation of prior symptoms.

Many factors govern the response of the patient after hysterectomy. These are:

- **Patient's age:** Older women are said to be more adaptable. Younger women in the third and fourth decades of life have fewer and less flexible coping mechanisms.
- **Socioeconomic status:** Women belonging to those strata of society that consider fecundity a measure of productivity, may show more tendency to develop depression. These women have not yet developed the self-image of being economically productive within the culture.
- **Indication for hysterectomy:** Hysterectomy done for benign indications has more psychologic morbidity than that for malignant conditions. This is because in a malignant illness, the affected organ is seen as a threat to life and its removal will bring a sense of relief and a new lease of life.
- **Preoperative mental condition:** Women who are less secure about their feminine identity, or more concerned about childlessness, may show a greater morbidity after genital surgery than women who are well adjusted to their sexuality and have completed their families. Significant post-surgical depression is seen in women who were depressed prior to surgery.
- **Oophorectomy:** It was found that women in whom the ovaries were preserved had better sexual adjustment than those who had oophorectomy. This effect was seen even in women who received oestrogen replacement after oophorectomy.

QUALITY OF LIFE

- Gynaecological disorders such as myoma uteri, endometriosis, pelvic pain and heavy bleeding are common phenomena. These conditions mostly cause discomfort and inconvenience rather than threaten life. They may, nevertheless, have an immense effect on a woman's quality of life (QoL) or on many aspects of her daily life, on her general health or sense of well-being, and produce a diversity of symptoms.
- When non-surgical management fails to resolve the suffering, hysterectomy is often performed to relieve symptoms and enhance the woman's QoL. Hysterectomy is one of the most frequently performed major surgical procedures and, therefore, its consequences concern a large number of women.
- Although recent studies have manifested positive outcomes after hysterectomy, concerns about the appropriateness of the operation have been heightened by reports of problems following the procedure. Thus, research has produced contradictory results concerning women's experiences following hysterectomy.
- Until recently, clinicians have tended to rely on objective measures in assessing the effects of medical interventions, and research has focused on the medical necessity of a procedure without examining the patient's perspective. Most trials, including that of hysterectomy as a medical treatment, have not measured QoL as a key outcome variable. Consequently, there has been little information from clinical trials

and prospective cohort studies on the effectiveness of hysterectomy for improving the QoL in women.

- Hysterectomy strongly improves general health to a level where it equates to that of the normal population. Persistent poor health among some hysterectomized women is mostly caused by factors other than the operation, such as responsibilities for caring for family members, occupational problems, as well as pain and other diseases.

- Recent research has, regardless of the use of different definitions and assessments, shown an enhancement in QoL and symptoms, during the early years after hysterectomy. These findings can be understood in the light of the problems gynaecological disorders generate. The pain, irregularity, heaviness and fatigue associated with menstrual disturbances may profoundly interfere with the highly valued active and independent lives most of the women in modern societies wish to lead. The inconvenience generated by these conditions creates a gap between the women's expectations and achievements, causing dissatisfaction with the areas of life that are important to them.

- The concerns that existed for years that hysterectomy could result in postoperative psychiatric morbidity were based on retrospective reports of high rates of depression, psychiatric referrals, and psychiatric hospitalizations in women undergoing hysterectomy. However, in the past decade, more rigorous and methodologically advanced studies have established that hysterectomy for benign disorders does not cause depression and may actually decrease psychiatric symptoms in many women and enhance their psychological wellbeing.

- However, studies have consistently found that presurgical psychopathology is predictive of postsurgical psychopathology. Thus, hysterectomy does not seem to cause psychopathology, but for women with a psychiatric history, the operation might be 'the straw that breaks the camel's back'. Previous abuse experiences might be related to persisting problems experienced by some hysterectomized women.

- Studies conducted over the last 30 years show that the majority of retrospective studies reported an adverse psychological outcome after hysterectomy, while all prospective studies showed that the incidence of depressed mood is higher even before the hysterectomy. Hysterectomy itself is not the cause of any adverse psychological outcome. Psychological symptoms actually improve in the majority of women. On the other hand, hysterectomy may not be of any benefit in women with a prior psychiatric illness and those with personality and psychosocial problems.

- The overall research evidence, therefore, shows that neither women awaiting hysterectomy nor those already hysterectomized suffer more psychological disturbances than other women. In previous studies, normal grief reactions after the loss of the uterus might have been interpreted as depression. Thus, an adequate 'mourning time' must be allowed before investigating psychological wellbeing in hysterectomized women.

- The uterus is a symbol of reproduction, and women may see themselves as defeminized by having a hysterectomy, but literature indicates that this surgery does not necessarily make the subjects feel any less a woman. If the woman's life work and sense of identity come from her childbearing role, hysterectomy can invoke a symbolic loss of purpose, even if it is performed after the menopause. However, in contemporary society, the de-feminizing effect of hysterectomy may be decreasing because the role and position of women in society have been changing, with a diminution in the importance of the motherhood role.

- Studies show that very few women regard the uterus as essential to their sense of femininity and womanhood. This could be understood in terms of the new female role, where an active life and control over one's own life is highly valued. The elimination of symptoms associated with abnormal menstruation—including irregular bleeding, anaemia, pelvic pain and pressure—allow the woman to re-enter society and establish an active, social and normal life.

- The role of the woman's partner in her reactions after a hysterectomy has been highlighted. A supportive and empathic partner can alleviate negative psychological reactions in a woman having a hysterectomy. Prehysterectomy relationship problems tend to predict further negative development of the relationship after the surgery.

- Men may feel confused when confronted with their partners' hysterectomy. The issue of a man's sexual life may be paramount in a situation where the woman has gone through a hysterectomy. Both women and men seem to need comprehensive information prior to and after this medical intervention. There is a scarcity of research on these matters in lesbian relationships.

MANAGEMENT

- Keeping in mind the main reason for a hysterectomy would help a woman in coping better with the recovery. A lot of women are uncomfortable with the prior medical condition that posts the surgery their lives improve.

- Talking to a psychotherapist will help them managing their thoughts, work on anxiety, depressive symptoms and accept the present situation.

- Having a support system will lessen the external burden of the woman. Supportive friends and family will help in psychological and physical recovery.

- It is important to make the patient understand that uterus was only a part of body that a woman has and not everything that makes her a woman.

- In order to understand women's reactions after the performance of hysterectomy, it is important for doctors and nurses to recognize all the factors that affect women's experiences. Some of these factors are partner relationships and support provided by the partner. Women undergoing hysterectomy express a need for information for both themselves and their male partners.

- From that point of view, efforts must be directed to the community to enlighten men and families about hysterectomy as a medical intervention by dispelling myths and providing current health information related to women. Women's QoL might be enhanced after a hysterectomy. Likewise, this medical intervention can also have a positive effect on the QoL of the male partners, since the women's suffering before the intervention may have a negative impact on their partners' QoL.

- Counselling programmes which target women and their partners together are recommended. The women's partners may present prevailing supportive attitudes and adequate reactions concerning the women going through a hysterectomy.

- For a woman facing the prospect of undergoing a hysterectomy, she mostly has enough time to investigate her priorities and values in life before actually deciding whether a hysterectomy is the best option for her. If she values a free, independent and active lifestyle highly, her choice might be different from that of a woman whose self-esteem is embedded in the notion of being fertile. The issue of age for the outcome of hysterectomy is not clearly understood.

- Further studies are needed before we fully understand how a hysterectomy can affect a woman's QoL and psychological health. There is also a need to illuminate the relationship between different surgical procedures and the patients' QoL. Studies are also needed to identify risk factors for developing a poor QoL after a hysterectomy.

RECOMMENDED READING

1. Bernhard LA. Consequences of hysterectomy in the lives of women. Health Care Women Int 1992;13(3):281–91.
2. Farrell SA, Kieser K. Sexuality after hysterectomy. ObstetGynaecol 2000;95(6):1045–51.
3. Khastgir G, Studd JW, Catalan J. The psychological outcome of hysterectomy. Gynecol Endocrinol 2000;14(2):132–41.
4. Rannestad T. Hysterectomy: Effects on quality of life and psychological aspects. Best Pract Res Clin ObstetGynaecol 2005;19(3):419–30.

Psychological Issues in Menopause

Komal Chavan, Avinash De Sousa, Meenakshi Ruhil

INTRODUCTION

Women form an important basis of the family and the society; thus society's health depends on the health, cultural, and economic needs of women. Women have a large number of duties and fulfillment of those duties requires complete physical and mental health. Menopause is one of the most critical phases of the women's life. The attainment of menopause makes women to undergo various physical, mental and psychological changes and a lot of such experiences which she has never went through. Menopause is defined as the permanent cessation of menstrual cycles for at least a year. Physiologically, menopause occurs due to the fluctuations and decline in the ovarian hormones. The mean age of menopause is between 50 and 52 years. However, it may vary from 44 to 54 years.

PATHOPHYSIOLOGY

Several hormones in the hypothalamic-pituitary-ovarian axis are indicators of ovarian aging, including FSH, oestradiol, inhibin B and AMH. FSH is secreted by the anterior pituitary and is regulated through negative feedback by inhibin B and oestradiol, hence an "indirect measure". As inhibin B and oestradiol vary through each menstrual cycle, FSH levels fluctuate accordingly. With ovarian aging, lower inhibin B also results in decreased negative feedback to the pituitary, resulting in increased FSH secretion and higher early follicular FSH.

With decreasing ovarian follicles with advancing age, both AMH and early follicular inhibin B levels decrease. Oestradiol is produced by granulosa cells of ovarian follicles in response to FSH stimulation. With ovarian ageing, oestradiol levels fluctuate and finally declines in menopause.

Pathophysiology of Psychiatric Disorders in Menopause

- Female reproductive hormones and rapid changes in their levels may influence neurotransmitters in the brain, particularly the serotonin and gamma aminobutyric acid systems. Oestrogen modulates serotonin to increase serotonin presynaptic reuptake, modulates norepinephrine levels, decreases monoamine oxidase levels, affects dopamine turnover, increases brain excitability, affects endorphin levels, and possibly interacts with gamma aminobutyric acid.
- Progesterone is found to increase monoamine oxidase levels. In high doses, progesterone has an anaesthetic effect and may decrease brain excitability through an interaction

with the gamma aminobutyric acid system. The drop in oestrogen levels during perimenopause and menopause can lead to hot flashes that disturb sleep. This can lead to anxiety, fears, and mood swings.

- The greater frequency of symptoms during the years prior to the end of the menses and the reduction of symptoms once menopause has occurred suggest that emotional symptoms are related to changing hormone levels rather than low hormone levels.
- Some women experience anxiety and depression, but women who have a history of poor adaptation to stress are more predisposed to the menopausal syndrome. The two most common psychiatric conditions are anxiety and depression.

Symptoms

- Irregular periods
- Vaginal dryness
- Hot flashes
- Chills
- Night sweats
- Sleep problems
- Mood changes
- Weight gain and slowed metabolism
- Thinning hair and dry skin
- Loss of breast fullness

Diagnosis

- Serum FSH
- Serum oestradiol

PSYCHOLOGICAL PROBLEMS IN MENOPAUSE

- Menopausal transition is phase of increased mental health problems in a woman, especially depression.
- Depressive symptoms during the menopausal transition could represent the recurrence of pre-existing psychiatric disorders or reflect a general vulnerability to develop mental health problems during stressful life events.[1]
- Persons who score high on neuroticism are more susceptible to the negative effects of daily stress and critical life events.[2]

Risk Factors for Developing Depressive Symptoms in Menopause[3]

- History of depression
- Vasomotor symptoms
- Sleep disturbances
- Surgical menopause
- Young at menopause
- Negative attitudes about ageing
- Life stressors

Role of Oestrogen in Psychology during Menopause

- "Hypoestrogenism hypothesis" proposes that gonadal dysfunction may increase vulnerability to schizophrenia, or that schizophrenia may lead to gonadal dysfunction.
- The "oestrogen protection hypothesis" proposes that oestrogen may play a protective role in women from schizophrenia, and may be a factor in the delayed onset of schizophrenia compared with men, less severe psychopathology, better outcomes, and premenstrual and postmenopausal deterioration in women.

Management

Hormone Replacement Therapy

- With the exception of the 0.14 mg ultra-low dose oestradiol patch, all systemic oestrogen formulations are approved for treatment of vasomotor symptoms.
- In women with intact uterus, oestrogen is given with progesterone to prevent the endometrial hyperplasia.
- Oestradiol skin patch is the most common transdermal formulation.
- Common adverse effects of oestrogen include breast tenderness, bloating, and uterine bleeding, which can be prevented by giving low dose oestrogen.
- **Indications:** Treatment of vasomotor symptoms and prevention of osteoporosis.
- **Contraindications:** *Absolute*: Unexplained vaginal bleeding; liver dysfunction or disease; history of deep venous thrombosis or pulmonary embolism, untreated hypertension; history of breast, endometrial cancer, history of CHD, stroke, or TIA.
- **Vaginal oestrogen:** For treatment of genitourinary atrophy.
- Calcium and vitamin D supplements to treat osteoporosis.

TREATMENT OF MENTAL ILLNESS DURING MENOPAUSE

- Antidepressants are the first-line treatment for menopausal mood disorders and anxiety disorders.
- In perimenopausal women with menopausal depressive disorder, there may be an indication for adjunctive therapy with transdermal E2 in refractory cases; oestrogen may augment the effects of selective serotonin reuptake inhibitor (SSRI) antidepressants as well as hasten the onset of antidepressant action.[4]
- Oestrogen also may be worth considering in women with mild depressive symptoms.
- For menstrual depressive disorders, SSRIs plus oestrogen may be more beneficial in improving mood than either agent alone.
- Venlafaxine improved the psychosocial domain, while oestrogen improved quality of life in other domains.
- Escitalopram, duloxetine, and citalopram have also been identified as having a possible positive impact on menopausal symptoms.
- SSRIs and serotonin-norepinephrine reuptake inhibitors may help reduce hot flashes and improve sleep.[5]
- Selective oestrogen receptor modulators (SERMs), such as raloxifene, which cause a tissue-specific E2 receptor activation and have less oestrogen-related adverse effects.[6]
- Therapy may focus on accepting a role transition and coping with loss of fertility.

- Cognitive behavioural therapy may be helpful for menopausal symptoms, including hot flashes, as well as depressive symptoms.
- Lifestyle modifications and exercise.
- A healthy diet, low in fat, high in fibre, with plenty of fruits and vegetables and whole grain.

REFERENCES

1. Nelson HD. Menopause. Lancet 2008; 371:760–70.

2. Mroczek DK, Almeida DM. The effect of daily stress, personality, and age on daily negative affect. J Pers 2004; 72:355–78.

3. Sajatovic M, Friedman SH, Schuermeyer IN, et al. Menopause knowledge and subjective experience among peri- and postmenopausal women with bipolar disorder, schizophrenia and major depression. J NervMent Dis 2006;194(3):173–8.

4. Dennerstein L, Soares CN. The unique challenges of managing depression in midlife women. World Psychiatry 2008;7(3):137–42.

5. Vivian-Taylor J, Hickey M. Menopause and depression: Is there a link? Maturitas 2014; 79(2): 142–6.

6. Kulkarni J, Gavrilidis E, Wang W, et al. Oestradiol for treatment-resistant schizophrenia: A large-scale randomized controlled trial in women of child-bearing age. Mol Psychiatry 2015; 20(6):695–702.

Psychological Issues in Gynaecological Cancers

Niranjan Chavan, Avinash De Sousa, Sneha Venkateswaran

INTRODUCTION

Cancer is one of the leading causes of disease in the world. The worldwide burden of cancer is estimated to be 14 million new cases per year. This number may rise to approximately 22 million in the next 20 years.[1] Gynaecological cancer is a common type of cancer. There is uncontrolled growth of abnormal cells originating in the female reproductive organs, including the cervix, ovaries, uterus, fallopian tubes, vagina, and vulva. Each cancer has its own set of risk factors, signs and symptoms, prevention and treatment modalities. A diagnosis of cancer can be emotionally and psychologically challenging and the needs of every patient must be addressed properly.

Cervical cancer is the fourth most common cancer in women all over the world. It is the second most common cancer in women living in regions that are less developed. World Health Organization (WHO) estimated approximately 570,000 new cases of cervical cancer globally (estimations for 2018), with approximately 318,000 deaths (representing 7.5% of all female cancer deaths). More than 85% of these deaths occurred in low- and middle-income countries.[3]

In India cervical cancer is the second most common cancer among women (Table 15.1).

Cervical cancer is a public health problem and account for one quarter of the worldwide burden of cervical cancers. It is the one of the leading causes of cancer

Table 15.1: Incidence of cancers among women in India[2]	
Site	Age-adjusted ratio
Breast	25.1
Cervix	21.2
Ovary	6.7
Oral cavity	6.4
Oesophagus	5.5
Stomach	3.4
Gallbladder	3.2
Leukaemia	2.9
Lung	2.7
Corpus uteri	2.5

mortality, accounting for 17% of all cancer deaths among women aged between 30 and 69 years.

The prevalence of endometrial cancer and hyperplasia was 1.0% and 5.8% in women of reproductive age and 3.0% and 12.1% in postmenopausal women, respectively. Being postmenopausal increased the risk of endometrial hyperplasia and cancer, while being postmenopausal and morbidly obese further increases the risk. No increase in risk was found in women of reproductive age who were either overweight or obese.

Ovarian cancer is the sixth most commonly diagnosed cancer among women in the world, and causes more deaths per year than any other cancer of the female reproductive system.[3]

PSYCHIATRIC COMORBIDITIES IN PATIENTS WITH CANCER

Psychiatric Comorbidities in Ovarian Cancer

The prevalence studies show depression (37.9%) (10–25%) and anxiety (29.8%). Within 2 months after cancer diagnosis, there was a peak in the overall incidence of mental disorders.[4] Among the mental disorders, maximum incidence was seen in stress reaction and adjustment disorders. Depression was seen more in patients of age group less than 60 years (40.4%). Anxiety was more in the age group of more than 60 years (39.4%). Age was a significant predictive factor for mental disorders, patients over 50 years were at a higher risk for mental disorders. Most commonly seen is depression, adjustment disorder and depression second to medical condition.

Aetiology and Pathophysiology

- Poor perceived social support
- Increased intrusive thoughts
- Younger age
- Inflammatory cytokines like IL-6 involved in tumour genesis
- Cortisol dysregulation

Clinical Features

- More vegetative features
- Fatigue
- Low psychomotor activity
- Greater functional disability

Psychiatric Comorbidities in Endometrial Cancer

Worldwide, endometrial cancer is the sixth most common cancer among women.

Causes associated with increased endometrial cancer incidence:

- Changes in childbearing methods
- Use of hormone-replacement therapy
- Aging population
- Reduced physical activity

Patient mortality can be increased as psychological problems may lead to poor compliance to treatment.

A Korean database showed depression and anxiety were diagnosed in 2.45% and in 3.37% among total cancer patients. Previous studies have shown that cancer survivors have an increased risk of depression, anxiety, and stress disorders within the first year following a cancer diagnosis.

Causes of Psychological Comorbidities in Endometrial Cancer

- Radical hysterectomy
- Treatment fear
- Treatment-related side effects, such as lymphedema
- Urological symptoms
- Sexual problems
- Cancer recurrence or progression
- Patients' reactions to anaesthetics and painkillers
- The hormonal imbalance caused following ovary removal
- The fear of surgical complications together with the impending loss of fertility

There was more incidence of depression in young endometrial cancer survivors. In contrast, the ratio of anxiety was higher in older age groups.

Anxiety was the most common disease in the preoperative period and depression as most frequently observed in the postoperative period.

Studies showed depression (43.9%), anxiety (43.7%), and stress reaction/adjustment disorders (12.3%) to be common.

Cortisol variability which is suggestive of higher hypothalamic-pituitary-adrenal (HPA) axis activation may lead to emotional distress associated with hysterectomy.

Premenopausal women hysterectomy with salpingo-oophorectomy may induce premature menopause and fertility loss. This change in hormonal status may affect patients' mood and put them at risk of depression.

Vaginal dryness after hysterectomy may affect sexual well-being.

Clinical Features

Depressive features are secondary to the cortisol variability

- More vegetative features
- Fatigue
- Low psychomotor activity
- Greater functional disability.

Psychiatric Comorbidities in Cervical Cancer

Cancer of cervix is the third largest cause of cancer mortality in India.

The diagnosis of cancer is the cause of stress on any individual which relates both to symptoms of the disease and psychological meaning attached to cancer.

Psychiatric morbidity was detected in 55% of females diagnosed as carcinoma cervix.

Studies showed that 26–34% were diagnosed as major depressive disorder, 17–39% as anxiety disorder, 8% as adjustment disorder with depressed mood, schizophrenia was 31% and 4% as insomnia and suicidal ideations.

Causes of Psychiatric Comorbidity

- Cervical cancer survivors (CCS) have to deal with bowel and bladder changes
- Sexual dysfunction
- Treatment related menopause
- Loss of fertility
- Relationship problems
- Sexual function and reproductive ability may be permanently impaired after treatment for cervical cancer. This can be a significant predictor of depression and anxiety.

Due to the involvement of reproductive hormones, women are especially prone to develop anxiety and depression.

There is a significant overlap between psychiatric symptoms and cancer with somatic symptoms such as fatigue, pain, reduced sleep, appetite and concentration.

As can be expected, the diagnosis of cancer leads to many mood disturbances in patients. Women with pre-existing mood disorders, or those who perceive their illness as 'severe' are at highest susceptibility for these disturbances. Some patients use positive ways to cope, such as seeking social support and assistance from friends and family. These women have less anxiety and depression. But when they use avoidance, their moods worsen.

RESPONSES TO TREATMENT OF CANCER

Some of the emotional stress due to the diagnosis of cancer is in view of anticipation of difficult treatment. Treatment monitoring and follow-up of the patient may even require repeated examinations and laboratory investigations. All these add on to the physical, psychological, emotional and financial burden to the patient and her family (Table 15.2).

1. **Surgery:** Cancer patients require radical surgeries which compromise on their quality of life in the long run. Added to the difficult postoperative recovery, there is also the apprehension regarding completeness of surgical procedure and fear regarding recurrences. Postoperative vaginal dryness, shortening of vagina and associated sexual dysfunction, dyspareunia and altered orgasmic function are common symptoms experienced by these patients. Surgeries, like pelvic exenteration, are disfiguring and produce many functional problems with obvious sexual sequelae.
2. **Radiotherapy:** This is a common treatment modality in gynaecologic cancer patients especially those with cervical or endometrial cancers. Patients in the low-income

Table 15.2: Currently available modalities of cancer treatment
• Surgery
• Radiotherapy
• Use of radioactive substances
• Chemotherapy
• Hormonal therapy
• Immunotherapy
• Combination of either two (e.g. intraoperative radiotherapy)

group and those with lower formal education are at higher risk to be non-compliant with radiation therapy as this therapy requires long-term follow-up. They may refuse treatment, terminate prematurely or take fewer sessions than prescribed. There may also be anxiety due to expected vaginal discharge, bowel and bladder disturbances associated with radiotherapy.

3. **Chemotherapy:** There is a general fear among the people regarding side effects of chemotherapy like nausea, vomiting, alopecia, etc. Fatigue is also a common symptom noted by patients receiving chemotherapy or radiation. These issues may cause them to not complete the prescribed course of chemotherapy leading to treatment failures and subsequent psychological morbidity.

Interventions

Considerable research has been done to formulate interventions to benefit the patients suffering from the psychological morbidities arising from the diagnosis and treatment of a life-threatening disease like cancer. However, there is a need to construct training programmes for gynaecologists, surgeons, physicians, oncologists and intensivists in order to allow better dissemination of this information from the healthcare providers to the beneficiaries.

- Procedural information—to clearly explain the entire surgical procedure in the best possible language to the patient and her attendant in the language they best understand, using visual aids as needed.
- Sensory information—information about the actual sensations of the surgery or the preparatory events leading to it.
- Behavioural coping instructions, relaxation, hypnosis and emotion-focused interventions.[4]
- To significantly reduce anxiety, depression, and overall discomfort in patients, training in relaxation and guided imagery techniques can be given. This is especially useful in the patients who require radiation therapy.
- Disease and treatment information, detailed information and explanation about side effects and warning signs related to the use of various chemotherapeutic agents and collaborating with palliative care experts are proven to be of benefit to patients receiving chemotherapy.
- It cannot be over-emphasized that patients having pre-existing psychiatric illnesses need to be referred to psychiatrists for appropriate treatment, ideally, before any intervention is undertaken for treatment of the gynaecologic cancer.

CONCLUSION

Women diagnosed with cancers should be treated with utmost care and compassion. Usually, women after undergoing surgeries for a malignant condition have better mood adjustment than women undergoing surgeries for benign conditions. This is because a cancerous organ is seen as a threat to life. Factors such as patient's age, stage of the disease, completion of childbearing and presence of any pre-existing psychologic morbidities must be taken into consideration to predict their response to the surgery or chemoradiation. There is also need for focused intervention to address sexual dysfunction. Behavioural sciences help in resolving quality-of-life issues.

REFERENCES

1. Stewart BW, Wild CP. World Cancer Report 2014. Geneva: WHO Press, 2015.
2. Uma Devi K. Current status of gynecological cancer care in India. J Gynaecol Oncol 2009;20(2):77–80.
3. Coleman MP, Forman D, Bryant H, Butler J, Rachet B, Maringe C, et al. Cancer survival in Australia, Canada, Denmark, Norway, Sweden, and the UK, 1995–2007 (the International Cancer Benchmarking Partnership): An analysis of population-based cancer registry data. Lancet 2011; 377,127–38.
4. Steginga SK, Dunn J. Women's experiences following treatment for gynecologic cancer. Oncol Nurs Forum 1997;24:1403.

Special Situations

Psychological Aspects of Rape

Tejasvi Dave, Sushma Sonavane, Sneha Venkateswaran

Rape is an act that violates the honor and bodily integrity of a woman. It destroys her physical and mental composure and sends her into a deep emotional setback. Rape is one of the most common crimes against women and a serious national problem in India. There is a new case reported once in every 20 minutes. According to the National Crime Records Bureau (NCRB) 2013 annual report, 24,923 rape cases were reported across India in 2012.

DEFINITION OF RAPE

Section 375 of IPC defines rape as a criminal offence and states that a man is said to commit rape when he has sexual intercourse with a woman against her or without her consent or if she is a minor. Under Section 375 of IPC, a man is said to commit rape, if he:

a. Penetrates his penis, to any extent, into the vagina, mouth, urethra or anus of a woman or makes her to do so with him or any other person; or

b. Inserts, to any extent, any object or a part of the body, not being the penis, into the vagina, the urethra or anus of a woman or makes her to do so with him or any other person; or

c. Manipulates any part of the body of a woman so as to cause penetration into the vagina, urethra, anus or any part of body of such woman or makes her to do so with him or any other person; or

d. Applies his mouth to the vagina, anus, urethra of a woman or makes her to do so with him or any other person, under the circumstances falling under the seven descriptions.

- Against her will.
- Without her consent.
- With her consent but the consent was obtained by putting her or any person close to her in fear of death or of hurt.
- With her consent but the man knows that he is not her husband and the consent was given because the woman believes that he is the man with whom she is or believes herself to be lawfully married.
- Consent given by reason of unsoundness of mind, or under influence of intoxication or any stupefying or unwholesome substance.
- With her consent but at the time of giving such consent the woman was unable to understand the nature and consequences of her consent.
- With or without her consent, when the woman is below the age of 18 years.

Consent

Consent means actively agreeing and clearly communicating to be sexual with someone. Consent should be freely given and can be taken away anytime. An individual also has the right to remove the consent during the sexual act.

What is NOT a consent: Silence, a forced 'yes', past consent, flirting, being unconscious, clothing or a maybe. Not fighting the act does not mean that consent is given.

Stigma

Stigma refers to the disgrace and negative beliefs associated with a particular thing. Along with physical and mental trauma, the victim has to deal with the added shame arising from the stigma. People often fail to realize that the comments, judgment, perceptions would affect the survivor. It indirectly implies that the survivor is in some-way responsible for the rape. A lot of times, the survivor is blamed for being raped. A rape is never a victim's fault. Stigma can multiply the pain and stops the victim from reaching out to others and seeking help.

AFTERMATH OF THE RAPE

- Along with physical consequences, rape also has long lasting and very often lifelong psychological consequences. These symptoms may or may not occur immediately. Soon after the incident, an individual may act in an unusual way, be withdrawn, communication may reduce, be fearful and emotionally unstable.
- A survivor may develop anxiety symptoms including excessive worrying, muscle tension, overthinking, suddenly going blank and phobias.
- Dissociation can occur during or after the assault.
- Post-traumatic stress disorder (PTSD) is also noticed where a person will have recurring nightmares, flashbacks, sleep disturbances and startle response.
- Depressive symptoms have been reported in almost all the survivors where there is excessive sadness of mood, hopelessness, increased or decreased appetite, isolation, insomnia or hypersomnia, somatic complaints, loss of energy, recurrent thoughts of death. Risk of suicidal ideations or attempts is high.
- A lot of survivors turn to psychoactive substances to seek temporary relief from the pain they are experiencing like alcohol or drugs.
- An individual may suffer from sexual dysfunction including chronic pelvic pain, dyspareunia and menstrual irregularities.
- Some of the individuals also report memory disturbances and cognitive distortions.
- Self-esteem reduces and sense of identity is questioned.
- A survivor may also develop the symptoms of paranoia, suspiciousness and trust issues.
- Childhood and adulthood victims of sexual assault are more likely to attempt or commit suicide.

Other consequences that a survivor could face are gynaecological disorders, reproductive disorders, infertility, pelvic inflammatory disease, HIV/AIDS, chronic pain, unwanted pregnancy and its complications.

All the above symptoms may result in the interpersonal conflicts with friends and family, marital disharmony, conflicts at workplace, difficulty in communication with the male gender and decrease in the work performance.

Clinical Intervention

Early intervention is critical for sexual assault victims because the level of distress immediately following the assault is strongly correlated to future pathologies. The intervention consists of pharmacotherapy and psychotherapy.

Pharmacotherapy

SSRIs like fluoxetine, sertraline, escitalopram and fluvoxamine are effective in treating PTSD and major depression. Antidepressants like mirtazapine and desvenlafaxine are also useful. Short-term use of benzodiazepines like clonazepam and lorazepam are helpful to control anxiety features.

Psychotherapy

- Social acknowledgement is very important in the healing process. Society has to accept that an individual is suffering. A lot of factors like news on media, harassment on the roads, sex are constant reminders of the horrifying incident that took place. A lot of individuals are in denial and refuse to reach out due to factors like stigma, self-doubt, guilt, shame, fear and if the offender is known. Healing is a painful process and requires proper support.
- Along with the medicines to manage the symptoms, psychotherapy, social support groups, family and friends can help in managing the survivor.
  - The aim of psychotherapy would be to help the client accept the incident, manage the thoughts, help in adjusting socially, reduce the anxiety, PTSD and depressive symptoms.
  - Along with the improvement in the mood and anxiety, it helps in building self-confidence, self-esteem, improve communication and expressions, strengthen inter-/intra-personal relationships and improving the judgement.
- Social support groups are a place where a survivor would come across people who have been through a similar incident. An individual may find this place very safe and secure. A person feels that she is not the only one and reduces the feeling of isolation. Everyone in the group supports one another, thus instilling hope. It also improves the interpersonal relationships and coping strategies.
- Family and friends can do a number of things that will help the survivor like:
  - Believe whatever they say
  - Don't judge
  - Reassure that it was not their fault, give them the time they need
  - Help them gaining confidence
  - Give them privacy for a while, if the need
  - Help them gaining control over the life
  - Treat them as survivors and not the victim
  - Have empathy but don't display pity
  - Constantly motivate them to continue with the treatment and also be a part of the process wherever necessary
  - Do not ask them to move on
  - Be careful of what and how you speak

Rape is a crime driven by the need to control, humiliate and harm. It is a petrifying act that changes an individual forever. The proper management techniques and social support would help the survivor to recover and heal.

MYTHS AND FACTS RELATED TO RAPE

There are certain myths regarding rape that need to be clarified:

1. **Rape is a sexual act:** Rape is not in fact a sexual act but rather is pseudo-sexual act. It is a sexual act for non-sexual needs. It is an act to manifest domination and express hostility where sex occupies a secondary position.
2. **Rape is an act of impulse:** Most rapes are often premeditated and carefully planned though not all may be so. Most studies have found when surveying criminal records that only 16–20% of rapes are ones which have occurred spontaneously.
3. **Rape occurs only among strangers:** It is very often seen that in many cases the rapists know their subject prior to the rape. Often rapists are close friends and even members of the family including distant relatives.
4. **The victim was in some way party to the offence:** It is often felt that the victim was asking for the rape, provoked it or was seductive or provocative. Victims may be women that are elderly, children, fully clad and even rape of nuns has been reported. Very often an innocent victim is the one that is raped.
5. **If she really wanted, the woman could prevent rape:** The fact is that most of time rape occurs through intimidation with a weapon, threat of harm or injury and even via brute force. Different motives operate in different offenders and they may use different ways to make the victim submit to them.
6. **Women make false allegations:** It is often felt that women make false allegations to take revenge on the accused. In fact, many women that are raped by men they know do not report to the police as they do not wish to be questioned about the rape and do not wish to see themselves as rape victims. In fact, cases of sexual assault and rape are grossly under reported as per official records.

THE TYPES OF RAPE

1. **The adult rape:** This is the rape of a young woman that the assailant likes due to proximity or certain special characteristics. It is not uncommon to find that the victim has been spurning the love attempts of the assailant which continue to the fateful day when the assailant takes full advantage of the prevailing circumstances either in the hope of succeeding in his amorous exploits by forcing the victim to comply and rape being a punishment for non-compliance.
2. **The child rape:** This may vary from an infant to an older girl that attends primary school to a much older girl in her teens. A minor girl may be threatened and offered certain benefits and forced into certain situations. She may give into the assailant due to ignorance. Children that pursue attention seeking behaviour, use their eyes and limbs and freely touch any stranger unknown to them often the ones that are involved.
3. **The college girl rape:** This is often seen in a teenager that may proceed into a sexually compromising situation either after being drugged or may be raped by her partner while she does not comply for the completion of the sexual act with a partner that cannot control himself at this juncture.

4. **The retarded girl rape:** Very often mentally retarded girls who are ignorant and keep quiet are the victims and very often for days no one knows about the incident until an accidental pregnancy is detected.
5. **War rapes:** These are situations where rape is used as a method of exercising control over a defeated nation. Rape in warfare is a planned strategy as well as an impulse motivated act geared towards the complete demoralization of the defeated side.
6. **Gang rape:** When more than two assailants are involved in raping a single victim then the phenomenon is termed a gang rape.

THE PROFILE OF THE RAPIST

1. **The power rapist:** Here for the rapist, rape is a means by which he reassures himself of his sexual adequacy and manhood. The rape is pre-meditated and preceded by an obsessional fantasy of victim resistance which he finds highly desirable. Such a rapist may be inadequate in negotiating interpersonal relationships and sexual as well as non-sexual areas of his life. The victims usually lie in his own age group.
2. **The anger rapist:** Here the anger rapist expresses his anger, rage, contempt using typical brutality. His aim to vent his anger against women and to retaliate against the rejections that he suffered against the hands of women in the past. These rapists often find no sexual satisfaction in rape and anger is the sole motive.
3. **The sadistic rapist:** Here both sexuality and aggression become fused into a single experience called sadism. The offender finds maltreatment of his victim intensely gratifying and may subject the victim to abusive acts like biting and burning certain specific body parts or sexual areas.
4. **The child rapist:** This is often seen in rapists that have a feeling of inferiority and a child is selected for the act as there shall be less resistance from the victim to the assailant.
5. **The alcoholic rapist:** Here rape is committed by a rapist that is under the influence of alcohol and controls are lost and consciences are quelled likewise. These are people that often get strong sexual urges under the influence of alcohol and if no outlet is provided, they resort to rape to fulfil their urge.
6. **The mentally ill rapist:** Here rapists commit rape as part of abnormal mental process where can hardly be held responsible for the rape when it occurs. They are often very aggressive. In certain extreme situations, they may even commit murder after rape. Certain brain tumours in the temporal lobes of the brain may cause an intense sexual urge that may cause an individual to seek satisfaction via rape though these cases are extremely rare.

RECOMMENDED READING

1. Cohen LJ, Roth S. The psychological aftermath of rape: Long-term effects and individual differences in recovery. J Soc Clin Psychol 1987;5(4):525–34.
2. Weidner G, Griffitt W. Rape: A sexual stigma. J Personality 1983;51(2):151–66.
3. https://www.crimesolutions.gov/PracticeDetails.aspx?ID=18
4. http://lawtimesjournal.in/rape-and-its-punishments/

Psychological Aspects of Widowhood

Avinash De Sousa, Komal Chavan

INTRODUCTION

- Worldwide, widows comprise a significant proportion of all women, ranging from 7 to 16% of all adult women. In developed countries, widowhood is experienced primarily by elderly women, while in developing countries, it also affects younger women, many of them still rearing children.
- Women are more likely than men to be widowed for two reasons. First, women live longer than men and women tend to marry older men, although this gap has been narrowing.
- Widowhood presents a myriad of economic, social and psychological problems, particularly in the first year or so after the death of the spouse. A major problem for both sexes is economic hardship. When the husband was the principal breadwinner, his widow is now deprived of his income and the nucleus of the family is destroyed.
- Widows have higher mean levels of traumatic grief, depressive and anxiety symptoms (compared to widowers) as well as have higher levels of mental illness than the general population.
- An important problem associated with widowhood is loneliness. Many widows live by themselves. They suffer the fear of being alone and loss of self-esteem as women, in addition to the many practical problems related to living alone.
- The greatest problem in widowhood is still emotional. Even if it had been a bad marriage, the survivor feels the loss. People respond differently to loss and overcome grief in their own time. Frequently, the most difficult time for new widows is after the funeral. Young widows often have no peer group. Compared to older widows, they are generally less prepared emotionally and practically to cope with the loss.
- There has been considerable controversy as to whether widowhood is a more difficult experience psychologically for men or for women. Widowhood is generally a greater problem financially for women than men, and economic difficulties can lead to lower psychological well-being.

WIDOWHOOD IN INDIA

- India has the largest recorded number of widows in the world, i.e. 33 millions (10% of the female population, compared to only 3% of men), and the number is growing because of HIV/AIDS and civil conflicts. 54% women aged 60 and over are widows and 12% women aged 35–39 are widows.

- India is perhaps the only country where widowhood, in addition to being a personal status, exists as a social institution. Widows' deprivation and stigmatization are exacerbated by ritual and religious symbolism.
- Widow remarriage may be forbidden in the higher castes; and remarriage, where permitted, may be restricted to a family member. Further, a widow, upon remarriage, may be required to relinquish custody of her children as well as any property rights she may have. If she keeps her children with her, she may fear they would be ill-treated in a second marriage.
- Indian widows are often regarded as "evil eyes", the purveyors of ill fortune and unwanted burdens on poor families.
- Many widows are disowned by their relatives and thrown out of their homes in the context of land and inheritance disputes. Their options, given a lack of education and training, are mostly limited to becoming exploited, unregulated, domestic labourers (often as house slaves within the husband's family), or turning to begging or prostitution.
- Younger widows are often forced into prostitution, and older ones are left to beg and chant for alms from pilgrims and tourists. Older widows may have lived the greater part of their lives in these temples, having been brought there as child widows many years before. The ordeals of the temple widows and the occasional sati are publicized in the international press.
- Widows, through poor nutrition, inadequate shelter, lack of access to health care and vulnerability to violence, are very likely to suffer not only physical ill health but stress and chronic depression as well.

PSYCHIATRIC ASPECTS OF WIDOWHOOD

- A large number of studies have been done focusing on the psychiatric aspects after death of the spouse. Depressive episodes were common after the death of a spouse. A high index of suspicion should be maintained by clinicians for the possibility of depression, particularly in cases of the young widows and widowers with such a history.
- Those who experience depressive symptoms soon after the loss may better be considered to be suffering from depression than bereavement. Researchers have noted the existence of subsyndromal symptomatic depression contributing significantly to morbidity in widows and widowers during the first 2 years of bereavement.
- Widows must be assessed for depression rather than viewing altered behaviour among the bereaved as socially or culturally acceptable, psychological aspects too should be considered. The predisposition to develop anxiety as well as substance abuse disorders also increases after widowhood.
- Widowhood and divorce are significantly distressing events in the life of an individual, with associated psychological ramifications. These problems are further compounded among women owing to particular social and cultural aspects, which lead to increased feelings of guilt, remorse and aloofness.
- There is also a tendency to reject depressive symptoms as something socially and culturally acceptable, whereas significant distress associated with these events could be harbingers of psychiatric illness often requiring attention (medical or otherwise).

- NGOs and other such self-help groups who come to the aid of such women should be appraised of the possibility of such entities so that proper attention and early intervention can be initiated.
- It would also be beneficial, if women who themselves have undergone such an experience come forward to help others. This would serve the twin benefits of rehabilitating these women as well as providing the needed care and support to the distressed among them.

SOME OTHER FACTS

- Widowhood is associated with a multitude of adverse physical and mental health outcomes including psychological distress, physician visits and institutionalization, and higher rates of morbidity and mortality. Prevalence rates of clinical depression within the first year of widowhood are estimated between 15 and 30% across studies, though subclinical elevation in depressive symptoms is even more common.
- Although depressive symptoms diminish over time among the widowed, they seem to remain high for many years following widowhood, at least in comparison with married persons in cross-sectional studies.
- Men and women experience widowhood at different stages of the life course, which in turn leads to diverging consequences with respect to their psychological well-being. Some widows and widowers are "transient" (i.e. they remarry or die soon after), whereas others may spend decades widowed. In other words, we have to distinguish between the short-term bereavement effect on psychological well-being and the long-term effect of widowhood as a marital status.
- The widowed population is highly heterogeneous with respect to the timing and duration of widowhood.
- There is a duration effect, whereby men's shorter widowhood duration leaves them less time to adjust, so they appear more vulnerable compared with women who have been widowed longer.
- There is a timing effect, whereby women's selection into early widowhood results in higher vulnerability compared with men, if indeed early widowhood leads to more adverse outcomes. The timing effect does not state that women are necessarily more vulnerable to early widowhood than men, but simply that more women than men enter widowhood through this pathway.
- Compared with men, women are more likely to become widowed at an earlier stage of the life course and to remain widowed for a longer period of time; second, early widowhood is associated with poor psychological well-being that does not seem to improve over time.
- The effects of early widowhood are substantial and chronic for those who remain widowed, whereas those widowed at later ages are more likely to recover, at least in terms of depression. Future research would do best to focus on gendered pathways to widowhood, rather than on gendered outcomes of widowhood.

RECOMMENDED READING

1. Carr D, Utz R. Late-life widowhood in the United States: New directions in research and theory. Ageing Int 2001;27(1):65–88.

2. Raveis VH. Facilitating older spouses' adjustment to widowhood: A preventive intervention program. Soc Work Health Care 2000;29(4):13–32.
3. Scannell-Desch E. Women's adjustment to widowhood: Theory, research, and interventions. J PsychosocNursMent Health Serv 2003;41(5):28–36.
4. Trivedi JK, Sareen H, Dhyani M. Psychological aspects of widowhood and divorce. Mens Sana Monogr 2009;7(1):37–45.
5. Umberson D, Wortman CB, Kessler RC. Widowhood and depression: Explaining long-term gender differences in vulnerability. J Health Soc Behav 1992;1:10–24.
6. Zisook S, Shuchter SR. Major depression associated with widowhood. Am J Geriatr Psychiatry 1993;1(4):316–26.

18

Psychological Issues in Lesbians

Pragya Lodha

INTRODUCTION

Lesbians are a sub-group of the LGBTQ+ community, defined as females having a homosexual orientation where they are romantically and/or sexually attracted to females. The LGBTQ+ community being a minority and discriminated group of individuals, they face social ostracization, stigma and negative attitudes and it is documented that they also face 2-3-fold higher mental health problems than their heterosexual counterparts. Within the LGBTQ+ community, lesbians and *trans* persons are the further discriminated group, who have to face challenges in addition to that the community faces.

Before we discuss the psychological issues that lesbians face, it is important to understand the history which will help us to better understand the roots of the continued discrimination against lesbians.

Homosexuality was considered to be a mental disorder till 1973 and it was only after the publishing of the *Diagnostic and Statistical Manual of Mental Disorders III* (1978) that it was formally derecognized as one, however, the stigma against the homosexual persons has persisted over decades. Arising from the label of a mental illness, several gay men were coerced into treatment for 'rectifying' their orientation. The scenario for lesbian women was somewhat like this: Some women actively sought help from the medical and psychiatric establishment. Most women who voluntarily sought help received some kind of psychotherapy from a range of practitioners, including psychiatrists. Some wanted an explanation of their sexual desires, others wanted help to be 'normal' and 'overcome homosexual tendencies' because of feelings of guilt and shame. These women presented to services in distress and despair because of struggles with their sexual orientation, isolation and social ostracism.

Records from 1965 disclose that female homosexuality was understood as "a sexual neurosis and is just as treatable as any other neurosis" and psychiatrists claimed to have 'cured' a number of female patients through psychotherapy. Unpublished data has been found in the mid-1970s that suggests that small numbers of women were treated for 'sexual deviation' as their 'primary diagnosis'. There are instances of use of electroconvulsive therapy which were often reported as 'successful' in the literature, however, women reported that it made them feel 'terrible' for months, and that although it resulted in them not being able to act on their attraction to women, at least for a period of time, it did not make them more attracted to men. There are documentations of women being treated with lysergic acid diethylamide (LSD) in the 1950s and 1960s to "overcome their sexuality". There are isolated evidences for a woman receiving deep insulin coma treatment to treat her sexuality in the 1950s and a woman who was threatened with psychosurgery in the 1950s. A number of accounts describe women being treated punitively to induce shame because of their sexuality when they were psychiatric inpatients, including being segregated from other female patients.

PSYCHOLOGICAL ISSUES

The following are psychological issues that lesbians face and some other issues that challenge the lesbians and have psychological underpinning:

1. The prevalence of mental health problems among the LGBTQ+ is found to be 2-4-fold higher than their heterosexual counterparts. The delay in medical and mental health treatment has also found to be 2-3-fold higher.

2. There are bodies of research that show poor prediction of mental health for lesbians as compared to heterosexual women, however, there is also data informing us that they are only slightly more likely than heterosexual youth to attempt suicide, refuting previous research that suggested much higher rates.

3. There are common research findings that tell us about low self-esteem and low well-being reported among the homosexual women. However, in contrast, a study found lesbians reported equally strong levels of mental health as their heterosexual sisters and higher self-esteem.

4. Higher rates of major depression, generalized anxiety disorder and substance use or dependence have been reported in lesbian youth.

5. People often assume there are less cases of violence in lesbian relationships because men are typically more violent and likely to be abusers. Domestic abuse is actually more common in lesbian relationships than heterosexual relationships and other groups within the LGBT spectrum—44% of lesbian women reported intimate partner violence compared to 35% of heterosexual women and 26% of gay men.

6. The process of coming out, by definition revealing one's sexual identity, is one that has seen decrease in age over the years, from the age of 20 in 1970s and 80s to the age of 14 in 2015. This poses psychological challenges as the younger cohort has lesser cognitive capability to deal with the societal stigma and discrimination which may be faced as a consequence to 'coming out'. There is a sense of loss that females report to experience socially and psychologically, which is clinically essential to evaluate as they raise the vulnerability to develop further mental health problems.

7. Being subject to homophobic attitudes and outright social distancing increases the risk for developing depression, anxiety and in many instances, increase the risk for suicide as well.

8. The pressure to identify and reveal oneself as a lesbian becomes a compulsion especially around heterosexual counterparts and among males. This may be distressing especially for those may not have come out or may not want to come out. There is no need for one to reveal their orientation unless warranted for, personally.

9. There are several assumption and stereotypes associated with being lesbian and often lesbians find themselves at the receiving end of humour and shame. The negative attitudes include: They hate men, they are more masculine than

heterosexual women, they have not met the right man, they dress like men, they are more interested in sports and that being with women is more of an experiment than a sexual preference.

10. It is a misnomer and derogatory to affirm the status of a woman being lesbian as a result of them having being abused by men in their childhood. This has a direct negative effect on the mental health of the female, sometime leaving long-lasting impact and leading to greater risk to mental illnesses as well.

11. Another factor that adds to distress is that lesbian relationships are conferred with a notion that one of the females has to take the role of a man to make the relationship meaningful; however, this is not true.

12. Lack of familial acceptance and societal support along with homelessness increases the mental health vulnerability for lesbians due to increased incidences of abuse, violence and maltreatment with little or no support.

13. Lesbians are also found to indulge in increased substance use as a result of unhealthy coping mechanisms against depression, anxiety, isolation and abuse.

14. There is an absence of dating culture and exclusion from prominent dating culture, for lesbians, in the LGBT community exacerbates the social isolation and anxiety lesbian women try to overcome. There is also the possibility that the lack of dating culture contributes to the problem of some lesbian women being too aggressive in establishing a relationship.

15. Another common challenge for lesbians is when it comes to parenting. By default, especially, in Asian cultures, lesbians are considered incapable parents for the lack of 'fatherly' nature in the lesbian relationships which make parenting and child-nurturing an incomplete process. However, this is not true.

How to Address Psychological Issues in Lesbians

The means of addressing psychological issues in lesbians take the course of common practice along with certain specific guidelines in place in order to take care of special challenges that arise in the lesbian population. The following are some points of management to aid the management of psychological issues among lesbians:

1. It is the responsibility of the mental health professionals to be aware of the sexual minorities and patients must not become a source of educating/psycho-educating the professional at the time of consultation. It is not only unfair to their time but also adds onto their stress and may sometimes be derogatory to the patient.

2. Professionals must strive to understand the effects of stigma—prejudice, discrimination, and violence—and its various contextual manifestations in the lives of lesbian population and how it exacerbates their mental and overall wellbeing.

3. One of the most important considerations for professionals is to fully recognize that being lesbian (and any other LGBTQ+ person) is not a mental illness. The professionals must have a homo-friendly attitude towards the patient, because only then will they be able to understand the problems of the patient with empathy which can guide to appropriate management of mental health problems.

4. It is also very crucial to remember that same-sex attractions, feelings and behaviour are normal variants of human sexuality and that efforts to change sexual orientation have not been shown to be effective or safe.

5. Professionals must make an effort to realize the uniqueness of the patients and build on them. This facilitates rapport and aids a better perspective of understanding the complaints.
6. Another crucial feature of understanding that plays role in understanding the nature of problems and addressing the problems is to be able to conceptually differentiate between sexual orientation and gender identity.
7. The ethical practices of equality, justice, fair treatment, beneficence and non-maleficence must be maintained.
8. The sociocultural factors such as religion, age, spirituality, socioeconomic class and other variables that are important at the intersection of identity along with the status of being lesbian must be acknowledged in treatment.
9. Identifying unique risks and challenges to the lesbian population makes for a helpful approach.

RECOMMENDED READING

1. American Psychological Association (2011). Practice guidelines for LGB clients: guidelines for psychological practice with lesbian, gay, and bisexual clients. *Washington, DC: American Psychological Association. Verfügbarunter: http://www. apa. org/pi/lgbt/resources/guidelines. aspx (Meldungvom 8.3. 2011).*
2. Baams L, Grossman AH, Russell ST. Minority stress and mechanisms of risk for depression and suicidal ideation among lesbian, gay, and bisexual youth. *Developmental Psychology* 2015;51(5): 688.
3. Coyle A, Wilkinson S. Social psychological perspectives on lesbian and gay issues in Europe: The state of the art. *Journal of Community & Applied Social Psychology* 2002.
4. D'Augelli AR, Pilkington NW, Hershberger SL. Incidence and mental health impact of sexual orientation victimization of lesbian, gay, and bisexual youths in high school. *School Psychology Quarterly* 2002; 17(2): 148.
5. DeAngelis T. New data on lesbian, gay, and bisexual mental health. *Monitor on Psychology* 2002; 33(2): 46–47.
6. Hafeez H, Zeshan M, Tahir MA, Jahan N, Naveed S. Health care disparities among lesbian, gay, bisexual, and transgender youth: A literature review. *Cureus* 2017; 9(4).
7. Koh AS, Ross LK. Mental health issues: A comparison of lesbian, bisexual and heterosexual women. *Journal of homosexuality* 2006; 51(1): 33–57.
8. Mustanski B, Andrews R, Puckett JA. The effects of cumulative victimization on mental health among lesbian, gay, bisexual, and transgender adolescents and young adults. *American Journal of Public Health* 2016; 106(3): 527–33.
9. Russell ST, Fish JN. Mental health in lesbian, gay, bisexual, and transgender (LGBT) youth. *Annual Review of Clinical Psychology* 2016; 12: 465–87. doi:10.1146/annurev-clinpsy-021815-093153.
10. Shearer A, Herres J, Kodish T, Squitieri H, James K, Russon J, Diamond GS. Differences in mental health symptoms across lesbian, gay, bisexual, and questioning youth in primary care settings. *Journal of Adolescent Health* 2016; 59(1): 38–43.

Psychological
Issues in Transgenders

Komal Chavan, Pragya Lodha

INTRODUCTION

A person's gender identity is their own sense of whether they are male or female, or neither. Some transgender people identify themselves with their changed gender: From male to female or female to male. However, others see themselves as members of a third sex. Officially now, the transgender is the third gender, in recognition and identity. 'Trans' is an umbrella term used for persons whose gender identity does not conform to their biological sex. The Indian population has more than 5 lakh individuals that belong to the trans community, one of the largest communities globally. Despite the Indian government's recognition of the transgender as the 'third gender' (NALSA judgment, April 2014), the trans community continues to face discrimination and is denied their fundamental rights such as access to education, workplace and healthcare.

Transgender people seek mental health care for various reasons apart from issues resulting from one's gender identity which could cause them distress or confusion. Some of the several mental health issues faced by the trans community apart from gender dysphoria, involve depression, post-traumatic stress disorder (PTSD), anxiety (social anxiety, specific phobias), bipolar disorder, schizophrenia, suicidal ideation, sexual abuse relationship dissatisfaction like in any other heterosexual or homosexual relationship issues, emotional health concerns and lack of sensitive, affirmative therapy among the trans community. Some of the psychosocial challenges for the trans community involve, lack of acceptance by family, gender identity confusion, homelessness, domestic violence and sexual harassment, bullying and being treated as an outcast. There are several other vulnerabilities identified in relation to health issues that further increase the likelihood of poorer mental health: A lack of safe environments, poor access to health services, challenges to the continuity of care-giving by their family and friends, and poor mental health resources. Feelings of shame and unworthiness have been found to be common among trans communities. While some may be seeking specific assistance for gender-related problems, others are seeking assistance with depression, anxiety, or other clinical concerns possibly unrelated to their gender identity. However, most of the mental health problems among the trans is concerned to do with how their identity is seen. In a transphobic society, discrimination for the trans begins with their appearance as it cannot be concealed.

PSYCHOLOGICAL CHALLENGES AMONG THE TRANSGENDERS

There are several challenges specific to the mental health of the trans persons that the community faces, especially so in the Indian scenario:

1. In the past, mental health issues for transgender people were narrowly viewed under the diagnosis of gender identity disorder. This led to pathologizing of the person's unique psychosocial experiences, therefore, limiting therapeutic responses and treatment options. The diagnosis of 'trans-sexualism' first appeared in the *International Statistical Classification of Diseases and Related Health Problems in 1975 and, in 1980, in the Diagnostic and Statistical Manual of Mental Disorders III.* However, recent research advancements (beginning since 2013) have confirmed that being transgender is not a mental illness. But in India, little medical research has been conducted on the issues of trans persons and the notion that being transgender is a mental illness continues.

2. Health care needs and social experiences vary across the lifespan. Identities for the young people often take shape by findings ways to integrate their identity into their cultural background, personal characteristics and family circumstances. Experiences of young transgender people continue to remain invisible and their concerns often neglected as they are always discriminated from the larger society. This hampers the emotional, social and cognitive development of the youth.

3. There is lack of psychoeducation among family members in order to understand the status of being trans which deviates from the heteronormative norms of the society. This further means that there is lack of sensitivity to the issues that trans individuals face and feel as individuals which further leads to an unwarranted divide among them and their family members. Overall, in the larger picture, this translates into lack of acceptance from the society, by large. The rate of homelessness is the highest among trans individuals.

4. On the other hand, families with children or family members belonging to the trans community have distinct and unique needs that fail to get met due to the lack of specialized care and trained professionals to address the same. For family member to settle with calling one of their children or family members with another pronoun (a boy who identifies with being female, may disclose at the age of 16 years that he would like to be addressed as 'she'), simply acknowledging that their child or member is willing to undergo sex transformation or simple day-to-day issues can sometimes get difficult in the initial phase.

5. Importance of informed consent, confidentiality and anonymity is equally important for everyone irrespective of their age, gender or any other socio-demographical feature. However, the larger clinical practice sees that though these norms are maintained for the heterosexual population, there is a compromise in following these ethical principles of practice when it comes to homosexuals or trans individuals as a consequence of the inherent bias that may be held against them.

6. Another concern that holds against trans patients is that there is greater stigma attached to approaching for help in a homophobic and transphobic society. Chances are less to find to a homosexual doctor or therapist as oppose to a greater chance of finding heterosexual professionals (though they may and most often, they do lack specialized care skills and knowledge to treat trans patients).

7. Not all trans adolescents have gender dysphoria or wish to undergo sex reassignment surgery, however, it is a commonly misunderstood paradigm where the dissonance between an individual's gender and sex is always looked at reconstructing and fixing them to align. On the contrary, another problem can arise, if an adolescent may wish to undergo the sex reassignment surgery where there may be two issues—one, either there is a confusion whether the teenager is sure enough for the surgery and second is the disagreement about the surgery between the adolescent and his or her parents.

8. There is no expert clinical consensus nor clinical guidelines regarding the treatment of prepubescent children who meet the diagnostic criteria for gender dysphoria. It is believed that gender dysphoria usually translates from adolescence to adulthood, however, such is not the case. It has been found that merely 6 to 23% of boys and 12 to 27% of girls treated in gender clinics have shown persistence of their gender dysphoria into adulthood.

9. There are several instances when children, adolescents and young adults have been taken to psychotherapists or counsellors by their parents with the notion that counselling can transform rather 'correct' their sexuality. However, these are myths and anybody who conforms to these practices in affirmation would be suspected on ethical (health care) practices. As opposed to this view, sex reassignment therapies are meant for those who wish to get themselves biologically corrected in order to conform to their psychological sex or the gender they wish to conform to (which is usually biologically the opposite).

10. The assessment before the sex reassignment surgeries and accessing hormone treatment remain at the merciful approval of the practitioners, some of them who continue to give a diagnosis of Gender Identity Disorder (the revision of Gender Identity Disorder in DSM IV TR has evolved to that of Gender Dysphoria in DSM 5 which implies the treatment of distress, depression or anxiety due to the non-conformity to the gender and does not involve any techniques or therapies to dissuade the personal choice/preference of an individual to identifying with a gender). The process of pre-counselling before the sex reassignment surgery may miss the underlying emotional factors and many a times, involves dissuasion room the sex reassignment surgery in order to conform to the biological sex of the individual. Ethically, before the surgery, the individual is made to undergo various social norms and make lifestyle choices so as to prepare them for the post-surgery life.

11. Post-surgery and post-hormone treatment care and counselling is missing, which is a crucial aspect in order to build and settle the transformations in the patient.

12. One of other nuances that often go amiss is the difference between sexual orientation and gender identity. Though the two are interlinked, they are different concept in existence and understanding. Professionals must be clear and precise about making of note of the same. When talking about sex reassignment surgery, it is important to know the gender identity of the individual and not the sexual orientation.

13. Unrequired electroconvulsive therapy (ECT), tying the patients to beds and institutionalization are resorted for convincing patients about the 'consequences of sex change' and instead stand the chance of an ethical dilemma. Unfortunately,

several practitioners resort to giving ECT in order to prevent the sex reassignment surgery for the individual thinking it is part of the treatment, however, one must be aware that this means is hoax.

14. As a result of the apparent stressors, an increasing number of transgender people are seeking therapy. However, therapists often lack the skills to work effectively with transgender clients and are often insensitive, ignorant and unaware regarding the several transgender issues. Many mental health professionals and medical practitioners lack an understanding of the LGBTQ spectrum health issues. Thus, an expertise to treat their concerns with an understanding of the ethical standpoints is missing.

15. The distinct needs of families with a transgender family member have often been neglected and children are increasingly in need of support. It has been clearly identified that access to family and couples therapy remains limited, if it exists in the first place. It transpires that most professionals in mental health services have received no training on transgender issues and there are visible shortcomings in terms of mental health education and curriculum developments. This denies the trans community the treatment they deserve. However, in the present times, the training for the same has taken a start but is a long way to go.

16. It has been noticed that practitioners harbour personal biases and prejudices in taking up trans patients for therapy or treatment. Psychiatrists and psychotherapists have a biased choice for taking up patients for treatment and thus may invariable deny the required and optimal mental health services needed by the trans individuals.

17. Counselling and psychotherapies also need a branch of specialization in order to understand and appropriately address the concerns and mental health issues of trans communities that are amplified due to multiple concerns. After having recognized the 'third' gender, the education and training centres fail to be inclusive in terms of providing the care for trans community.

How can Psychological Issues in Transgenders be Addressed?

Some very fundamental steps that can be taken up at an individual and societal levels in order to ensure a just status of the trans community are:

1. Gender dysphoria must be understood correctly that it is the underlying depression or distress due to gender confusion or social ostracization and not a pathological identity/personality.

2. Psychoeducation to one and all about the existing trans identities and their challenges should be addressed in order to ensure that the community acts in a sensitive manner towards them.

3. Health care settings must offer a safer environment for trans persons to bring up mental health concerns and should make access to mental health services easy for them. Every person taken as intake for primary health care concern should include a mental health history and an assessment for active mental health concerns. Screening should include for primary mental health problems, environmental and social stressors, and gender-related needs.

4. When there is a trans patient that a mental health professional is unable to handle, one must appropriately refer to transgender-affirming mental health services

where mental health professionals specialize in the field of LGBTQ+ mental health and thus will be more equipped to treat them.

5. Professionals should take the responsible effort of understanding the community and their specific challenges in healthcare.
6. There should be specialization courses run for treating individuals from the trans and LGBTQ+ community in order to better address their concerns and handle their specific mental health concerns with due sensitivity and responsibility.
7. School curriculums can also include to discuss the growing minority population and their challenges.

RECOMMENDED READING

1. Balakrishnan VS. Growing recognition of transgender health: stigma, discrimination and lack of legal recognition remain major barriers for transgender people to access the health services they need. Bull WHO 2016;94(11):790–92.
2. Benson KE. Seeking support: Transgender client experiences with mental health services. J Feminist Fam Ther 2013;25(1):17–40.
3. Deutsch MB (ed). Guidelines for the primary and gender-affirming care of transgender and gender nonbinary people. University of California, San Francisco; 2016.
4. Erickson-Schroth L (ed). Trans bodies, trans selves: A resource for the transgender community. Oxford University Press; 2014.
5. Lev AI. The ten tasks of the mental health provider: Recommendations for revision of the World Professional Association for Transgender Health's Standards of Care. Int J Transgenderism 2009; 11(2):74–99.
6. Lodha P. Better Mental Health Services for Trans-Persons in India-There is a Need for Understanding, Training and Infrastructure. [Internet]. January 21,2017. Available from http://newsnviews.online/news-n-views/better-mental-health-services-for-trans-persons-in-india-the-need-for-understanding-training-and-infrastructure/
7. Nagarajan R. First count of third gender in census: 4.9 lakh. The Times of India.2015 May 30. News India, [Newspaper on the Internet]
8. Richards C, Bouman WP, Seal L, Barker MJ, Nieder TO, T'Sjoen G. Non-binary or genderqueer genders. Int Rev of Psychiatry 2016;28(1):95–102.
9. Shipherd JC, Green KE, Abramovitz S. Transgender clients: Identifying and minimizing barriers to mental health treatment. J Gay Lesbian Ment Health 2010;14(2):94–108.

CHAPTER

20

Dementia and Women

Avinash De Sousa, Komal Chavan

- There is increasing attention to differences between men and women in the causes, manifestations, response to treatments, and outcomes of neurological diseases (dimorphic neurology). This attention to dimorphic medicine has historically been stronger in fields like cancer, cardiovascular diseases, and endocrine diseases.
- However, there is now a growing awareness of differences in brain structure and function between men and women throughout the entire life course (early childhood development, adult life, and aging). Second, there is increasing recognition of the distinction between sex and gender.
- Sex is biology: Chromosomal, hormonal, or reproductive differences between men and women. By contrast, gender refers to psychological, social, political, and cultural differences between men and women.
- It remains unclear whether women have a higher risk than men to develop dementia or Alzheimer's disease (AD) at a given age. Several European studies have suggested that women have a higher incidence rate of dementia or AD than men. However, studies in the United States have not shown a difference, or the difference has varied with age.
- Regardless of this difference in risk (in incidence rates) across continents, all studies consistently showed that more women than men have AD at any given age, possibly because women survive longer. This higher number of women affected may not be true for other types of dementia such as vascular dementia or Lewy body dementia.
- Limited attention has been given to the sex chromosomes in relation to the aetiology of diseases in general and of dementia or AD in particular. Women have two copies of chromosome X, one of maternal origin and one of paternal origin. The X-chromosome carries approximately 1,600 genes (approximately 155 million base pairs), including genes encoding the androgen receptor and several proteins involved with mitochondrial function, adipose tissue distribution, apoptosis, and response to hypoxia.
- There are risk factors that are equally common in men and women but have a stronger effect in one sex or gender group (e.g. APOE genotype). There are risk factors that have a similar effect in men and women but are more common in one sex or gender group because they are gender related (e.g. education). There are also risk factors restricted to one sex (e.g. oophorectomy).
- The E4 allele of the apolipoprotein E gene (APOE) is the strongest known susceptibility variant for AD. There are three major isoforms of the ApoE protein

(ApoE2, ApoE3, and ApoE4) that are encoded by three alleles of the APOE gene (E2, E3, and E4). Carriers of one E4 allele are three to four times more likely to develop AD than non-carriers. Carriers of the E4 allele also have an earlier age at onset of AD that can be visualized in cumulative incidence curves.

- Carriers of two E4 alleles have an even higher risk of AD than carriers of one allele (trend by genetic dose). The majority of studies, and a large meta-analysis showed higher age-specific odds ratios of AD in women compared with men both for carriers of one E4 allele and for carriers of two E4 alleles. Interestingly, the women to men differences were greater for carriers of one E4 allele than for carriers of two E4 alleles. The effect of the E4 allele was reduced after age 85 years in both men and women.

- Among E4 allele carriers, women showed greater hippocampal atrophy, more changes in the default mode connectivity, more cortical atrophy, and worse memory performance compared with men. In addition, a large autopsy study showed a higher burden of amyloid plaques and neurofibrillary tangles in the brain of women than of men who were carriers of an E4 allele. Finally, a recent study suggested that the greater risk of AD in women compared with men who carry one APOE E4 allele may be mediated by tau pathology.

- The stronger effect of the APOE E4 allele in women compared with men offers an excellent example of a completely biological factor (a genetic variant) interacting with other biological factors (e.g. hormones produced by the ovaries or other genes hosted on chromosomes X or Y) or with gender-related factors (e.g. education, physical activity, behavioural preferences, type of occupation). We will first describe possible interactions between APOE E4 and sex mediated by hormonal mechanisms.

- It has been postulated that the oestrogen produced by the ovaries in a woman before the onset of menopause has an important neuroprotective effect on the brain. The stronger effect of the APOE E4 allele on the risk of dementia in women may be mediated by oestrogen. Indeed, it has been hypothesized that the apolipoprotein E (ApoE: The protein coded by the APOE gene) may be a critical factor in the neuroprotective actions of oestrogen.

- Another line of reasoning for the differences between men and women focuses on possible interactions between APOE genotype and more conventional risk or protective factors for dementia or AD. APOE E4 genotype may interact synergistically with alcohol intake, cigarette smoking, physical inactivity, and high intake of saturated fat with the diet. These interactions may explain the increased risk of dementia and AD in APOE carriers in general. These interactions may also explain the differential effects of APOE genotype in men and women because men and women differ in their exposure to cigarette smoking, alcohol drinking, dietary preferences, and willingness to engage in physical activity.

- It remains unclear whether these behavioural factors are completely gender-related or whether they are partly biologically driven (sex related). It has also been suggested that higher education may reduce the harmful effects of APOE E4. Indeed, women who carried an APOE E4 allele had reduced risk of developing dementia, if they obtained a higher level of education early in life.

- Lower education is recognized as one of the most established risk factors for dementia and AD. Some studies suggested that the effect of lower education may be even stronger than the effect of the APOE E4 genotype.

- It remains unknown how education may prevent dementia and AD, and current data suggest that the impact of education on the risk of dementia or AD is similar in men and women. It may be strategic to consider education within a broader concept of intellectual enrichment that includes other protective activities or behaviours. It has been hypothesized that lifetime intellectual enrichment may provide an important brain reserve mechanism to delay the onset of cognitive decline and dementia.
- Education in earlier life (through schooling or formal training), mental stimulation as part of a job, and stimulating leisure activities later in life are three examples of factors that are primarily gender-related and historically contingent. In some countries, men had historically more access to advanced education than women; this pattern has now reversed.
- Oophorectomy and other gynaecological surgeries are examples of factors restricted to one sex because of anatomical differences. The neuroprotective effect of oestrogen may be lost in women who experience premature (before age 40 years), or early (between age 40 and 45 years) menopause either naturally or because of medical or surgical interventions (more commonly, bilateral oophorectomy).
- The risk increased with younger age at oophorectomy, did not vary by indication for the oophorectomy, and was eliminated by oestrogen therapy initiated after the surgery and continued up to age 50 years or longer. In most of the women, the bilateral oophorectomy was performed at the time of a hysterectomy.
- Earlier age at surgical menopause was associated with faster decline in global cognition, and specifically in episodic memory and semantic memory. Earlier age at surgical menopause was also associated with increased AD neuropathology, in particular neurotic plaques.
- Oestrogen therapy that was initiated within 5 years of the surgery and that was continued for at least 10 years was associated with a slower decline in global cognition. None of these associations were observed for women who underwent natural menopause.
- It has been suggested that bilateral oophorectomy causes an abrupt decline in the levels of circulating oestrogen, and that this decline may trigger a chain of causality leading to degenerative and vascular lesions in the brain. These brain lesions may manifest as cognitive impairment or dementia several decades after the oophorectomy. The role of other ovarian hormones (e.g. progesterone) and of other aetiologic mechanism (e.g. disruption of the hypothalamus-pituitary-ovarian axis) remains uncertain.
- Similarly, the effects of hysterectomy on the remaining two ovaries, or the effects of removing one ovary on the single remaining ovary are unknown. If the major mechanism linking bilateral oophorectomy with cognitive impairment or dementia is oestrogen deprivation, we must postulate that oestrogen is neuroprotective in women before the age of natural menopause.
- Hysterectomy, unilateral oophorectomy, and bilateral oophorectomy are examples of sex-specific conditions restricted to women. Similar sex-specific conditions have been investigated less frequently in men. For example, it remains unclear whether men who are treated for prostate hypertrophy or prostate cancer have an increased risk of dementia.

RECOMMENDED READING

1. Azad NA, Al Bugami M, Loy-English I. Gender differences in dementia risk factors. Gender Med 2007;4(2):120–9.

2. Bamford SM, Walker T. Women and dementia-not forgotten. Maturitas 2012;73(2):121–6.

3. Proctor G. Listening to older women with dementia: relationships, voices and power. Disabil Soc 2001;16(3):361–76.

4. Rocca WA, Grossardt BR, Shuster LT, Stewart EA. Hysterectomy, oophorectomy, estrogen, and the risk of dementia. Neurodegen Dis 2012;10(1-4):175–8.

5. Ruitenberg A, Ott A, van Swieten JC, Hofman A, Breteler MM. Incidence of dementia: Does gender make a difference? Neurobiol Aging 2001;22(4):575–80.

Substance Abuse in Women

Avinash De Sousa

Reasons for gender differences in drug abuse are not yet clear but could have important implications for the development of substance abuse treatment interventions and programmes. The recent prevalence rates indicate that the number of female drug abusers is increasing, and the number of clinical studies in which sex and gender differences in drug abuse are investigated is steadily increasing.

DEMOGRAPHICS AND CLINICAL CHARACTERISTICS

- Several demographic and clinical factors that differentiate women from men with regard to substance use have been identified. Women are more likely than men to come from families where one or more members are also addicted to drugs or alcohol, attribute the cause of substance abuse to genetic predisposition, family history, or environmental stress, and attribute their drinking to a traumatic event or stressor.

- Additional research indicates that women who are addicted have a history of over responsibility in their families of origin and reportedly have experienced more disruption in their families than their male counterparts. Women are also more likely than men to be in relationships with drug-abusing partners or spouses who are drug abusers and to identify relationship problems as a cause for their substance abuse.

- In addition to interpersonal stressors, women are more likely to experience affective disorders, whereas men who are addicted are more likely to engage in sociopathic or criminal behaviour. Although many women support their habits through prostitution or petty larceny, men are more likely to rely on robbery, con games, and burglary to support their substance abuse.

- Several differences between older male and female alcohol abusers have been reported. Women are likely than men to be widowed or divorced, to have had a problem drinking spouse, to have experienced depression, and to report more negative effects of alcohol.

- Older women have later onset of alcohol problems, more vulnerability to addiction stigma, greater use of prescribed psychoactive medications, and are more likely to abuse multiple substances. Women are more likely to combine their prescription drug abuse with marijuana, cocaine, or other drugs. Investigators also find that women may view substance abuse more negatively and that the social stigma attached to the substance dependence may act as a deterrent for women, leading them to obtaining their drugs from legitimate sources such as physicians.

- These factors may have implications for understanding the effects of gender and widowhood on the development of late onset problem drinking. It is well documented that women face greater medical exposure to psychotropic drugs than men, but little research examines whether women also have increased use of prescription drugs with abuse potential.
- Data about women's abuse of or dependence on prescription medications are virtually non-existent. This is significant considering that women, particularly midlife and older women, are the largest consumers of prescription painkillers, antidepressants, and benzodiazepines.
- Clinical evidence reported in the literature suggests that prescription drugs, especially benzodiazepines, sedatives, and hypnotics, are frequently prescribed for and abused by older women. Older women are prescribed benzodiazepines more than any other age group. Age-related changes in drug metabolism, interactions with other prescriptions, and over-the-counter drugs and alcohol contribute to greater risks for cognitive impairment, dementia, and falls.
- Women incarcerated for drug-related offenses represent one of the fastest growing populations in jails and prisons. Statistics reported that they committed their offenses under the influence of drugs or alcohol.

BIOLOGICAL DIFFERENCES

- Research suggests that men and women differ in their biological and subjective responses to abused drugs. Women initiate cocaine use sooner, take less time to become addicted to cocaine, and report less euphoria and dysphoria compared to men.
- Women and men given equal doses of cocaine experience the same cardiovascular response despite the fact that blood concentrations of cocaine did not rise as high in women as in men. In studies involving long-term cocaine users, women and men showed similar impairment in tests of concentration, memory, and academic achievement following sustained abstinence, even though women in the study had substantially greater exposure to cocaine.
- Women cocaine users also were less likely than men to exhibit abnormalities of blood flow in the brain's frontal lobes. These findings suggest a sex-related mechanism that may protect women from some of the damage cocaine inflicts on the brain.
- Biological indicators point toward clear differences between men and women in the metabolism and other physiological effects of alcohol. Women become intoxicated after drinking smaller quantities of alcohol than men and achieve higher blood alcohol concentrations. Retrospective reports from alcoholics reveal that women consume lesser amounts and are less likely than men to drink daily or to engage in binge patterns of alcohol use. This may be related to the fact that women have less total body water than men of comparable size, meaning that they achieve higher blood alcohol concentrations than men after drinking equivalent amounts of alcohol.
- Important gender differences also exist in the physiologic effects of nicotine. Women and men are equally likely to become addicted to nicotine, yet women typically smoke cigarettes with lower nicotine content than those smoked by men, smoke

fewer cigarettes per day, and inhale less deeply than men. Females report positive mood increases to a greater extent after nicotine smoking and show a great decline in positive mood during smoking abstinence than men.

- Research is beginning to show that the progression, or developmental stages, of drug involvement is not identical for men and women. In the progression from legal drug use to illicit drug use, e.g. cigarette smoking plays a relatively larger role for women than for men, and alcohol use plays a relatively larger role for men than for women.

- Studies of self-quitters find that women are less likely to quit initially or to remain abstinent at follow-up. Possible explanations for this sex difference have been suggested, such as women's greater concern about weight gain, greater difficulty with negative mood (and higher prevalence of affective disorders), greater need for social support to quit smoking, and the effects of cigarette advertising targeted at women.

- The progression to dependence, particularly alcohol-use disorder, also seems to be different for women than for men. The interval between the age of first drinking and treatment-seeking tends to be shorter for women than for men. In addition, women progress between landmarks associated with the developmental course of alcoholism (e.g. regular drinking or loss of control) sooner than men.

- These findings have led to the theory that 'telescoping' may occur in women. This theory posits that there may be a shorter timeframe for the development of medical consequences and behavioural and psychological factors characteristic of an alcohol dependence disorder.

- With regard to initiation into illicit drugs, data suggest that women are more likely to begin or maintain cocaine use to develop more intimate relationships, while men are more likely to use the drug with male friends and in relation to the drug trade.

MEDICAL PROBLEMS IN FEMALE SUBSTANCE ABUSERS

- Women who abuse drugs have been found to get sicker more quickly and suffer higher rates of liver problems, hypertension, anaemia, and gastrointestinal disorders than male drug users. Women also experience gender-specific medical problems as a result of their addiction, such as a higher risk for infertility, vaginal infections, repeat miscarriages, and premature delivery.

- Despite lower levels of alcohol intake and shorter periods of drinking, women suffer more severe medical consequences than men, including liver cirrhosis. Postmenopausal women who drink moderate to heavy amounts of alcohol also have other health problems, including breast cancer. They are at higher risk for breast cancer and heart disease even if the amount they drink is less than that of their male counterparts.

- Women who chronically abuse alcohol have death rates 50 to 100% higher than men who have the same alcohol use patterns. Some research suggests that the impact of a given amount of smoking on lung cancer risk may be greater among women than men, and that exposure to environmental tobacco smoke may be associated with increased risk for breast cancer.

- Particularly alarming is that women may be at even greater risk than men for smoking-related diseases, including lung cancer and myocardial infarction. Men have higher prevalence rates of chronic obstructive pulmonary disease than women, which has been attributed to the historically higher rates of cigarette smoking in men.

- The interplay of gender-specific drug use patterns and sex-related risk behaviours creates an environment in which women are more vulnerable than men to infection with the human immunodeficiency virus (HIV). Women using intravenous drugs are at higher risk than men for acquiring HIV. Women are more likely than men to inject drugs, use drugs with many partners, share paraphernalia with an injection partner, exchange sex for money or drugs, and have difficulty negotiating condom use with their sex partners.

PSYCHIATRIC PROBLEMS IN FEMALE SUBSTANCE ABUSERS

- It is well established that women with substance abuse disorders present for treatment with significant psychiatric co-morbidity. Women show higher rates of certain co-occurring psychiatric disorders compared to men, such as major depression, social phobia, post-traumatic stress disorders and eating disorders.
- Gender differences in depression are generally thought to be related to the interaction of biological and psychosocial factors. Higher rates of depression occur among women who are poor, less educated, welfare-dependent, and unemployed.
- Gender differences in the relationships between depressive symptoms and drinking behaviour have been reported in problem drinkers, indicating that depression can play a dual role, at least for women. More specifically, if men and women are motivated to stop drinking, depression can trigger a change in the beginning of treatment of both genders.
- Studies of comorbid psychiatric disorders in opiate and cocaine abusers have shown higher percentages of affective and anxiety disorders in women than in men. In a recent study of treatment-seeking opiate abusers, lifetime psychiatric comorbidity was more than twice as common in women compared with men.
- Women dependent on methamphetamine are more likely to report depression, suicidal ideation, and a need for psychiatric assistance than men. Increased risk for depressive symptoms was observed for both women and men reporting methamphetamine dependence compared to those not reporting dependence.
- Another area of particular importance for women is substance abuse and victimization and violence. A growing body of evidence suggests that interpersonal stress and relationship conflicts are major triggers for relapse among women in drug treatment and that intimate partner violence may result in continued drug use and relapse.
- With the aging of the drug using population, a majority of women in substance abuse treatment are perimenopausal or menopausal. Risk factors for a more complicated menopausal transition (e.g. alcohol, smoking and illicit substance use, medical comorbidities, HIV/AIDS and hepatitis, premorbid and current psychological distress, few social and economic resources, and negative life events) are fairly widespread in substance abusing women.

TREATMENT ISSUES

- Women are underrepresented in substance abuse treatment programmes. In the admissions to substance abuse treatment programmes were women, but the ratio of women to men with dependence on illicit drugs is larger. Research indicates that women seek treatment for substance abuse less often than men.

- The low rates of substance abuse treatment entry among women may reflect the specific barriers they face. Barriers for young women that have been documented in the past two decades include pregnancy, lack of services for pregnant women, fear of losing custody when the baby is born, or fear of prosecution, voyeurism, and sexual harassment.

- Women seeking treatment have been found to have more substance-related problems, and those problems tend to be more severe than those of men entering treatment. For instance, women are more likely to encounter difficulty with transportation to treatment sites, inadequate health insurance, poverty, dealing with a relationship with a drug-abusing partner, and being less likely than their male counterparts to have someone actively supporting them in treatment.

- Treatment entry for men seems to be facilitated by social institutions such as employers or the criminal justice system, whereas for women treatment entry more often results from social work referral, suggesting that contact with social agencies eases women's entry into treatment.

RECOMMENDED READING

1. Ashley OS, Marsden ME, Brady TM. Effectiveness of substance abuse treatment programming for women: A review. Am J Drug Alcohol Abuse 2003;29(1):19–53.
2. Greenfield SF, Back SE, Lawson K, Brady KT. Substance abuse in women. Psychiatr Clin 2010;33(2): 339–55.
3. Tuchman E. Women and addiction: The importance of gender issues in substance abuse research. J Addictive Dis 2010;29(2):127–38.

Consultation Liaison of Psychiatry and Obstetrics and Gynaecology

Niranjan Chavan, Avinash De Sousa, Pragya Lodha, Meenakshi Ruhil

INTRODUCTION

- Psychiatric conditions not only exert their toll in terms of suffering, loss of function and poor quality of life, but also may complicate the diagnosis, treatment and prognosis of the medical surgical reason for admission.[1]
- Consultation-liaison psychiatry (C-LP) is the discipline model established to address the above problems.
- Consultation psychiatry mimics other consultation activity between different medical and surgical professions.
- Most consultation models are more doctor centred than patient centred.

ENHANCING GYNAECOLOGISTS' ALERTNESS

- Joint gynaecological–psychiatric education programmes.
- Continuous medical educational programmes for obstetricians and gynaecologists are highly recommended.
- Gynaecology–psychiatry combined case conferences might also be a good way to enhance gynaecologists' alertness toward mental illness in their patient populations.

REASONS FOR PSYCHIATRY CONSULTATION

- **Obstetric:** Depression and dysthymia were the most common diagnoses in obstetric inpatients referred for psychiatric consultation.[2] The second most frequent diagnosis was schizophrenia and other psychoses.
- **Gynaecological oncology:** Depression, anxiety and adjustment disorder.[3]

Evaluation

- Psychiatric evaluation in pregnant women requires careful evaluation of whether symptoms such as anxiety or depression are normative or pathologic, evidence of new onset of psychiatric disorder or of an exacerbation of a previously diagnosed, unrecognized or subsyndromal pre-existing psychiatric disorder.
- Physicians, therefore, should screen more intensively for psychiatric disorders antenatally, integrating questions about psychiatric symptoms and treatments into the comprehensive obstetric history.
- Unfortunately, routine screening for psychiatric disorders during pregnancy or the puerperium is uncommon.[4]

PSYCHIATRIC INTERVENTION

- Psychotropic medication is preferred over psychological intervention.[5]
- Psychological intervention might be difficult to deliver during patients' general medical hospitalization.
- Short-term supportive psychotherapy was the most frequent non-psychopharmacologic intervention.
- At the time of admission, the most frequently used psychotropic medication was benzodiazepine, which was also the most frequently recommended medication by the consultant.
- Antidepressants were the psychotropic medication most often recommended but not taken, with not only patients but also physicians concerned about antidepressant treatment in comparison with benzodiazepines.
- The main reason for fewer antidepressant prescriptions might be the consultee's clinical judgment (e.g. consideration of drug–drug interactions). But the real reason could not be identified in the present studies and should be investigated further.

CONCLUSION

- Present studies demonstrate a low referral rate for psychiatric consultation in obstetric and gynaecologic patients.
- Depression and past psychiatric history attracted physicians' attention most commonly, but other symptoms may be neglected.
- Psycho-oncology was the basis for the majority of psychiatric consultations in the obstetric and gynaecologic patients included in our study, a finding which indicates the need for more collaborative clinical work and research.

REFERENCES

1. Stewart DE, Lippert GP. Psychiatric consultation-liaison services to an obstetrics and gynecology department. CanJ Psychiatry 1988; 33:285–9.
2. Tsai SJ, Lee YC, Yang CH, Sim CB. Psychiatric consultations in obstetric inpatients. J ObstetGynaecol Res 1996;22:603–7.
3. Thompson DS, Shear MK. Psychiatric disorders and gynecological oncology: A review of the literature. Gen Hosp Psychiatry 1998; 20:241–7.
4. Cassem NH, Stern TA, Rosenbaum JF, et al. Massachusetts General Hospital Handbook of General Hospital Psychiatry. St. Louis: Mosby 1997;487.
5. Rigatelli M, Galeazzi GM, Palmieri G. Consultation-liaison psychiatry in obstetrics and gynecology. J PsychosomObstetGynaecol 2002; 23:165–72.

Index